Your Pocket Is What Cures You

Studies in Medical Anthropology

Edited by Mac Marshall

Your Pocket Is What Cures You

The Politics of Health in Senegal

ELLEN E. FOLEY

RUTGERS UNIVERSITY PRESS

NEW BRUNSWICK, NEW JERSEY, AND LONDON

LIBRARY OF CONGRESS CATALOGING-IN-PUBLICATION DATA

Foley, Ellen E., 1972–
    Your pocket is what cures you : the politics of health in Senegal / Ellen E. Foley.
        p. cm. — (Studies in medical anthropology)
    Includes bibliographical references and index.
    ISBN 978–0-8135–4667–4 (hardcover : alk. paper) — ISBN 978–0-8135–4668–1
(pbk. : alk. paper)
    1. Medical anthropology—Senegal—Saint-Louis Region.   2. Medical policy—
Senegal—Saint-Louis Region.   3. Public health—Senegal—Saint-Louis Region.
4. Medical care—Senegal—Saint-Louis Region.   5. Medical economics—
Senegal—Saint-Louis Region.   6. Saint-Louis Region (Senegal)—Social conditions.
7. Saint-Louis Region (Senegal)—Economic conditions.   I. Title.
    GN296.5.S38F65 2010
    362.109663—dc22   2009018768

A British Cataloging-in-Publication record for this book is
available from the British Library.

Visit our Web site: http://rutgerspress.rutgers.edu

Manufactured in the United States of America

To my parents for their longtime support,
to Ajayi who joined this work in progress,
and to my friends in Pikine and Mumbaay

CONTENTS

Acknowledgments   ix

1   A Different African Health Story   1

2   A Brief History of Senegal   20

3   Urban and Rural Dilemmas   37

4   Global Health Reform in Saint Louis   58

5   Market-Based Medicine and Shantytown Politics
in Pikine   84

6   Knowledge Encounters: Biomedicine, Islam, and
Wolof Medicine   96

7   Gender, Social Hierarchy, and Health Practice   115

8   Domestic Disputes and Generational Struggles
over Household Health   130

9   Encountering Development in Ganjool   143

10 Believe in God, but Plow Your Field   158

Notes   165
Glossary   169
References   173
Index   181

ACKNOWLEDGMENTS

As with any large project, many people and organizations contributed to the various research and production stages of this book. At Michigan State University I received support, assistance, and funding from the African Studies Center, the Department of Anthropology, the College of Social Science, and the Graduate School. The research for this project was funded by a U.S. Department of Education Fulbright-Hays Doctoral Dissertation Research Abroad Fellowship, a fellowship from the International Dissertation Field Research Fellowship Program of the Social Science Research Council with funds provided by the Andrew W. Mellon Foundation, and the National Science Foundation.

The Africanist community of professors and fellow graduate students at MSU greatly contributed to my development as a teacher and scholar. Bill Derman has been a wonderful mentor. His visit to Senegal in 1999 as well as his guidance throughout my career have provided invaluable encouragement and direction. David Robinson deserves special recognition for sharing his Senegal expertise and for convening the group of *senegalisants* in East Lansing. Cheikh Anta Mbacke Babou and Faatim Joob have been my fellow travelers in East Lansing, Dakar, Bawol, and Philadelphia. Cheikh has earned a special distinction for being an outstanding colleague, mentor, and friend.

In Dakar, Gary Engelberg provided strategic advice and tips for getting started. Issakha Jallo was instrumental in obtaining special research permission from the Ministry of Health. Aissata De and others at the Institut Africain pour la Démocratie offered friendship, logistical support, and a much-needed "office away from home" in Dakar. The Joob family has been a source of friendship, support, and humor over the past decade and a half. This research was inspired by Papa Joob's enthusiasm for Ganjool and his dedication to maintaining family ties across three continents. I want to offer very special recognition to the matriarch of the family, Ajaa Faatu Taal, who has extended countless kindnesses and courtesies to me over the years. Her courage and generosity are unparalleled, and she provided much of the inspiration for my interest in gender issues in Senegal.

This book would not have been possible without the openness and generosity of the women in Pikine and Daru-Mumbaay. They accepted me both as a friend, neighbor, relative, and anthropologist and always greeted my questions with enthusiasm. In Pikine members of the Xaal Yoon Wi women's association deserve mention as they made me an honorary member of the group and gave me a warm welcome at all group meetings and special events. Many fond moments were spent at the health liasions' tea-drinking sessions. Special thanks go to Maodo Jaagne for his assistance and to Mari Njaay and Gna Gna Jallo for their camaraderie and friendship. Madame Mbow of the Service Régional de Développement Communautaire was of tremendous help locating women's groups in Saint Louis and keeping me abreast of activities concerning women's issues.

The success of this project is also due in large part to the medical and administrative personnel of the Saint Louis medical district and the leaders of the Saint Louis health committees. It could not have been easy to have an anthropologist in their midst, but they accepted my presence and my questions with grace and humor. Many thanks to Papa Kumba Faay, Salif Dem, Abdul Aziz Njaay, Papa Musaa Faal, Ndey Fari Juuf, Abu Saar, and Sylvie Njaay. Mamadu Seck was of tremendous help understanding the internal politics of Pikine and the workings of the health committees.

One of the most important contributions to the research came from Abdulaay "Vieux" Gey who worked tirelessly as my research assistant and helped me navigate the winding footpaths in Pikine. The Xorom-Si association of Pikine offered assistance and support for this project as well as two enjoyable *yendoo* (afternoons) on the banks of the Senegal River. Thanks to the families of Lamin Gey, Marietu Joob, and Magette Joob, who continuously provided me with warm meals and warm conversation and truly became my extended family in Saint Louis. Tamsir Sylla proved his endless generosity by offering me housing and his friendship during my eight months in Saint Louis. A warm thank you to the Ndong family, particularly Mama and Ndey Awa for their friendship and camaraderie.

Perhaps the best part of my field research was the period when I lived in Daru-Mumbaay and was able to participate in the everyday life of the village. Thanks to my inner circle of friends and tea-drinking buddies Fanta Gey, Jaari Faay, Faatu Gey, and Khadi Jaagne. Special mention goes to Salla Faal for being the first to decide that she would be my friend. Khalifa Gey gets an award for best *attaya* (tea) and for being such an all around good sport. Kalla Joob was helpful with making maps and helping me navigate the political and social terrain of the village. Ajuma Ba and Faatu Gey helped me understand the context and contradictions of biomedical care in a village setting and helped with my demographic surveys. Faat Taal also helped with surveys and worked tirelessly as the only daughter in our household.

Sue Schneider was an extraordinarily generous and insightful reader in the later stages of preparing this manuscript. I can't thank her enough for the care and attention she gave to each chapter and for her tireless cheering from the sidelines. I'd also like to thank Craig Janes and the anonymous reviewer of the manuscript. I hope that I have done justice to their astute suggestions for revisions; any shortcomings are mine, not theirs. Thanks to Lexy Close for some eleventh-hour research assistance and for putting together the bibliography.

I would not have made it to the close of this decade-long project without the love, equanimity, and good humor of my husband, Ajayi Harris.

To all of those mentioned here and many more who contributed to this project in countless ways both large and small, *yall na leen yalla fey.*

Your Pocket Is What Cures You

1

A Different African Health Story

It was a clear, hot day in September, and in spite of the relentless sun my friend Faatu decided she wanted to visit Amadu, a well-known healer in a neighboring village known for his skill at *mocc*. After taking our bucket baths and getting dressed, we set out trudging along the sandy road to the *mocckat*'s house. We walked a few kilometers and arrived in the neighboring village and then found Amadu's house. His wives and several children were sitting outside in the court-yard. "Are you here for mocc?" asked one of his wives. Faatu nodded and the woman told us that Amadu was away but that we could go see his father instead. She pointed to a straw hut 20 meters from the main courtyard where we could find the senior mocckat.

We went to the older man's hut and repeated our series of greeting, "Have you spent the day in peace? Is all well in the house? Is all well with your family?" After I promised that I would learn more of the Pulaar language before our next visit, the healer asked Faatu to explain her problem. She responded that she had a lot of pain on her right side and shoulder. He began reciting phrases in Arabic in a low voice and then applied pressure to several points on her back and squeezed her shoulders in a form of traditional massage. After several minutes of shoulder and torso manipulation the treatment was complete. Faatu paid him fifty cents, and he told us to come back if the pain continued. "Did it work?" I asked her as we headed back toward the main road. She nodded and said it felt better.

When we got to the road we found another villager loading sacks of onions into a car to take to the market in Saint Louis, about 25 kilometers away. After some banter with the driver we convinced him to drop us off in Mumbaay on his way to town, and then we squeezed ourselves into the back seat in between the 50-kilo bags of onions. In all likelihood, Faatu's shoulder pain was the result of working on her own onion crop, which entails a daily routine of lifting bucket after bucket of water out of a deep well to water the fragile plants. With the arrival of the harvest, the most difficult period of the agricultural calendar was over, and Faatu and others could begin to recover from their intense work schedule.

When we arrived in Mumbaay we found our neighbor Rama weighing and bagging her small onion harvest as a dozen children from the neighborhood danced about and generally made a nuisance of themselves. I scooped up Fanta, Rama's four-year-old daughter, and slung her over my shoulder. "How much for this bag of onions? How about twenty-five cents a kilo?" The children dissolved in giggles and clamored to be the next sack of onions headed to market. The going rate for onions was indeed twenty-five cents a kilo, not a great price, but much better than the lows of five and ten cents a kilo in previous years. The onion crop would allow Mumbaay's farmers to pay their debts and to purchase several months worth of rice and cooking oil before they began once again to buy on credit. The most fortunate families would buy fabric for new clothing, and perhaps even seek medical care for the ailments they had neglected during the busy farming season. Until their crops were sold, villagers made the most of the limited medical resources available to them; their treatment decisions were greatly constrained by time, cost, and inability to leave their onion fields for more than a day at a time.

FOR THE PAST TWENTY-FIVE YEARS, the HIV/AIDS pandemic has dominated research, popular and academic publications, and global media reporting about public health in sub-Saharan Africa. Yet behind the dominant coverage of the continent's AIDS crisis lies an equally troubling reality: the story of increasing poverty, crumbling social services, and the redesign of health systems to shift costs and responsibility from African governments to their citizens. After two decades of structural adjustment lending programs, poor and middle-class residents of many African countries have limited access to even the most basic forms of health care. This decline in adequate medical care is the product of misguided economic policy; efficiency-driven economic reforms were accompanied by state withdrawal from social services, particularly health and education. In the neoliberal era, health systems have been transformed in order to reduce government spending in the name of achieving economic growth. Changes such as fees for services, generic drug sales, and community involvement in financial management of hospitals and clinics have been cornerstones of these reforms.

These changes to many African health systems came during a time when more and more people in the global South were struggling to secure basic necessities as unemployment soared and the prices of food staples and fuel increased. More than two decades into structural adjustment and privatization, which were designed to streamline economies and promote growth, many African economies continue to falter. Prices for basic goods continue to rise while purchasing power declines or remains stagnant. For Senegal's urban dwellers, allusions to "Article II" have come to symbolize the grim economic decline of recent years. Article II is the shortening of the national pastime, tea drinking, from three rounds of tea to two in light of ongoing economic scarcity.

Even in countries that have experienced economic growth in absolute terms, the growing gap between the rich minority and the poor masses has proven impossible to reduce. Senegal is no exception to continent-wide trends. Throughout the period of structural adjustment lending in the 1980s and 1990s, as growth in gross domestic product reached 5 percent in some years the absolute number of people living in poverty increased, as did the disparity between rich and poor (Duruflé 1994). While other regions of the developing world are being swept into the frenzy of transnational capitalism and global integration, much of Africa is experiencing "equally global forms of exclusion, marginalization, and disconnection" (Ferguson 2006, 41). The elusive promises of globalization offer constant reminders of the continent's inferior position in the world's economic hierarchy. While the poor citizens of many nations are frustrated that they are unable to reap the fruits of globalization, even more devastating is the decline in government health services.

Social scientists and other experts began to lament the near collapse of many African health systems by the mid-1990s (Turshen 1999; Schoepf et al. 2000). HIV/AIDS is just one manifestation of the ongoing crisis. For every HIV infection or death from AIDS-related complications there are dozens of invisible, quieter tragedies of maternal and infant death, childhood malnutrition, malaria, diarraheal disease, TB, and on and on. AIDS activists in the North and the South have rightly drawn attention to the global disparities in access to technologies for HIV prevention, testing, and treatment (Smith and Siplon 2006). But this surge of activist attention, thus far limited to distinct therapeutic constituencies such as the HIV positive or People Living with AIDS (PWLAs), draws little attention to problems of health infrastructure, access to primary health care, or other health-related resources. There are no activists marching against malaria, and little attention is paid to the "stupid deaths" that affect the poor in places like Senegal (Farmer 2005).

This book tells a different health story from the dominant narrative of the AIDS pandemic. It is the story of what is happening to ordinary men and women in Senegal who are precariously balanced on the twin precipices of crumbling health systems and economic decline. The central premise is that the problems and paradoxes of public health stem from the encounter between market-based health policies and local social and political systems that are rife with inequalities. I make the case that recent health reforms fail to accomplish their stated objectives, and they aggravate social inequalities in ways that have important implications for vulnerability to disease, health action, and health development. Although the book critiques the neoliberalization of global health policy, it is ethnographic in nature, for, "without ethnography, we can only imagine what is happening to real social actors caught up in complex microprocesses" (Marcus and Fisher 1986, 82). While economic shocks are often recounted in a language of aggregate statistics that captures stalled economic growth, rising inflation, devalued currencies, and stagnant GDPs, this book takes a community-level approach to illuminate the ways that social inequalities act as fault lines that shape individual experiences with larger socioeconomic crises.

From the beginning of this project I wanted to understand how global policies and their articulation in Senegal affect everyday life, and how anthropology might allow us to trace the links between the suffering of mothers and children in seemingly remote communities and the rise of neoliberal thinking in Washington and Geneva. Having seen firsthand the distress and sense of crisis taking root in the Senegalese countryside, I wanted an explanation of the profound disconnect between global health policies, governmental and nongovernmental (NGO) rhetoric about health and development, and the daily dilemmas unfolding in the rural and urban communities I have come to know over the past fifteen years. As I followed the processes of decentralization and the implementation of participatory management of health structures, I observed the tremendous influence of externally driven processes of change as well as the ways that local histories, politics, and social relations mediated the outcomes of these reforms.

The Research Setting

The site of this ethnography is the Saint Louis medical district in northern Senegal. The district encompasses the city of Saint Louis and the rural zone immediately surrounding it. Over a period of twenty months in the late 1990s, I followed the daily activities of the administrators and clinical personnel who were charged with making the citizens of Saint Louis their partners in health. I watched as battles for influence ensued between overzealous community leaders and recalcitrant nurses who were supposed to co-manage health clinic activities and finances. I listened to women complain about their limited access to health care, the poor quality of the care on offer, and their mistreatment by unsympathetic doctors and nurses. After many months I tracked down the head nurse of a neighborhood health post to get his side of the story of the dispensary's fall into bankruptcy. I witnessed the urgent and intimate household politics of therapeutic decision making in cases of serious illness, in which some individuals, particularly wives and mothers, were all but excluded from decisions about what would happen to sick family members.

As has come to be accepted in anthropology, every subject's perspective is partial and situated, and this book tells interlocking stories to capture a variety of vantage points from people living, working, and trying to stay well in Saint Louis. Within the Saint Louis district, the study focuses on one urban neighborhood, a shantytown called Pikine, and one village in the rural Ganjool region called Mumbaay. The perspectives and experiences of the medical district's frustrated administrators and clinical personnel, juxtaposed with the daily challenges of town and village residents, reveals the complexity of public health and managing illness. Much of the time, doctors and nurses could not elicit the behavior they desired from their patients, and patients were similarly disappointed with their medical encounters. The recent transition to a decentralized health sector and the reorganization of roles and responsibilities of patients, their families, communities at large, and medical personnel proved to be anything but smooth. Health reforms require new modes of operation and organization from medical personnel and patients alike. Yet these social actors reworked and transformed the policies as they were implemented in Saint Louis. Through the stories of tensions and conflict that health reform produced in rural and urban locations, this book provides a view of global development trends "from the inside out" as new ideas about how to run government health systems collide with the material, political, and social realities in Senegalese communities.

Although this book examines health reform from a fixed location in Senegal, it joins the larger body of scholarship examining changing trends in global health over the past twenty years. The social contract between states and citizens concerning the state's role in providing high-quality, low-cost primary health care has changed dramatically (Turshen 1999, 115). The rhetoric of primary care has survived the economic reforms of the last two decades, but there has been a fundamental shift away from the global promise of "health for all by the year 2000" made by the world's governments in 1978 at Alma Ata (Hong 2004). In exchange for access to basic clinical services and generic pharmaceuticals, citizens in most developing countries now pay user fees and purchase drugs at their local health post or medical center (Schoepf et al. 2000, 109; Turshen 1999, 48–52). Cost recovery is part of the new framework of participation in the partnership in health between the state and its citizens. Decentralization promises new mechanisms of accountability, but often leaves regional and municipal officials with full responsibility for their constituents with few resources to meet their needs (Turshen 1999, 55).

The changing arena of public health in Saint Louis sets the stage for an examination of how people manage risk, illness, and vulnerability in Pikine and Mumbaay. Using an analytic framework based in critical medical anthropology (CMA), this book highlights health practice by exploring how rural dwellers and urbanites conceptualize health resources, and it examines how social and material power influences individuals' ability to make use of those resources. Stories of what happens when people get sick highlight how vulnerability to disease and health strategies are mediated by social position and power within families. By looking at the things that people do or don't do when faced with illness, we confront the sharp divide between the logic of market-based medical care and the structural limitations on health action. Health systems are designed with the rational economic actor in mind, but health decisions are often constrained by household power relations, hierarchies of age and gender, and structural inequalities of class and geography.

While power and inequality are central to understanding health strategies, this book also examines how health dilemmas reflect the social production of health knowledge. Just as men and women infrequently behave as the rational, economic actors envisioned by health planners and policymakers, what they know to be true about health, illness, disease, and medicine is often not what biomedical clinicians want them to know. Whereas the Senegalese Ministry of Health and partnering NGOs promote biomedical frameworks for responding to disease and promoting health, health action results from encounters between Islam, biomedicine, and indigenous medical traditions. Health-related knowledge and practice are situated; understandings of health and the ability to act on these understandings are shaped by factors such as social location with households and family structures, education (or lack thereof), age, and economic status.

While the city of Saint Louis struggles with rapid, unplanned urbanization, the Ganjool region has experienced sharp economic decline and a rapid livelihood transition to migrant fishing over the past fifteen years. By paying close attention to health dilemmas and power relations within rural and urban families, we observe how social hierarchies and gender ideologies mediate the effects of broader socioeconomic change. These recent trends have put additional stress on traditional fault lines of gender, age, and generation, particularly in Ganjool, where older men are increasingly losing access to the labor of their male dependents at earlier and earlier ages. The illness episodes recounted in the later chapters of the book allow us to analyze gendered dimensions of power and differential access to social and economic resources, and how these in turn influence the therapeutic process. To unravel the social processes that constrain people's health actions, I explore overlapping arenas of power and influence in formal and informal spaces of household and family, the village, the neighborhood of Pikine, and the city of Saint Louis.

In spite of the recent dramatic changes in Senegal's government health system, health development work continues unabated. Health workers organize nutrition projects, international donors promote family planning and HIV/AIDS education, and child-sponsorship NGOs build schools and health huts in rural villages. Most of these health interventions operate with several tacit goals: to introduce new kinds of health resources (condoms, breast cancer screenings, birth control, health hut education sessions), to convince people that these new resources are valuable, and to ensure that people will use them. Much like Tolstoy's unhappy families, each of these initiatives fails in its own way. Yet most failures stem from the predictable tendency to overlook the material and sociocultural basis of health behavior. By looking at several thwarted attempts at health development in Pikine and Ganjool, the book offers an account of how these projects misread local contexts and produce unexpected and undesirable results.

Culture, Power, and Practice

Several contemporary trends in anthropology have shaped my intellectual trajectory as an anthropologist, and their influence is evident in my approach to the broad themes of gender, health, power, and culture. Since the pioneering work of Franz Boas in the nineteenth and twentieth centuries, American anthropology has tended to place culture squarely at the center of its analysis. Nonetheless, theoretical introspection and the resulting transformation of the field over the past thirty years have shifted both our understandings of culture and the place of culture in anthropological inquiry. My career began in the 1990s when two important feminist anthropologists, Sherry Ortner and Lila Abu-Lughod, were part of a larger conversation about remaking anthropology, particularly in terms of our understandings of culture, gender, and the importance of power and practice to social analysis. Ortner and Abu-Lughod provided my generation of anthropologists with new theoretical approaches to the nagging problem of structure and agency, and a new mandate for leveling the historical hierarchy between a Western self and a cultural Other that is inherent to traditional conceptualizations of culture.

Ortner's ongoing refinement of Bourdieu's practice theory charted new territory, a way for cultural anthropologists to engage with structural inequalities and power without losing sight of what she refers to as the "intentional subject" who was absent from the structure-driven analysis of the political economists and poststructuralists (Ortner 1984, 2006). Practice in Bourdieu's formulation is human action, but in particular practice involves strategic improvisations and interests that are pursued as strategies (Bourdieu 1977). These strategies unfold in a social context that is shaped by the varying interests of individuals and their competition for economic, social, and cultural capital. Building on Bourdieu and Giddens, Ortner (1984) argues that the goal of anthropological analysis is not to capture Culture writ large but practice, what people do and say in the world, with the goal of explaining the relationship between human action and the global entity. In its most ambitious cast, practice theory offers a way of analyzing the mutual influence of human action and the social world by assessing the role of human action in making and reproducing the system (the material and symbolic aspects of society), while acknowledging that human action can also dismantle and transform the system (Ortner 1984). While practice theory offers a way of engaging with human action, one should not assume too much action, as action always takes place in the midst of tensions and constraints.

Essential to my analysis here is how practice theory aims to reconcile the relationship between overarching social structures and the thinking, acting, strategizing (and to development planners, aggravating) subject. The individuals in this book are caught up in a variety of macrolevel processes largely beyond their control, from state reforms to the collapse of rural livelihoods, yet it seems impossible to ignore the ways they strive to get what they want, playing any number of interrelated "serious games," albeit not under the circumstances of their choosing. In the face of seemingly overwhelming obstacles, young men continue to migrate, mothers visit health clinics, and wives lobby husbands and in-laws for financial support. The serious games in Wolof society of gender, health, production and reproduction, and being a pious Muslim, to name a few, are still being played, but at the moment of this research they were unfolding against a backdrop of shifting political economies and significant changes in the health system.

My research began with a relatively simple empirical question: what were the effects of neoliberal economic policies and efficiency-driven health reforms on rural and urban communities in Senegal? After witnessing, thinking, and writing about dilemmas of illness and health in Senegal for over a decade, I find that the most useful questions seem to be not ones of cause and effect but of process and encounters, negotiation and mediation. In what ways has the changing political and economic terrain influenced therapeutic processes, and in what ways are these shifts themselves mediated through Wolof social structures? What can we learn about processes of social and economic change by focusing on the household politics of health and illness? This book attempts to answer these questions.

Although Ortner and other practice theorists succeeded in decentering culture from its starring role in American anthropology, there have also been important shifts in how the discipline conceptualizes culture. In "Writing against Culture," Abu-Lughod put forth a scathing critique of the traditional notion of culture, and she points the way toward a more reflexive and serviceable approach to culture (1991). She argues convincingly that anthropology's classic ways of approaching and understanding culture served as a tool of essentialism, a way to exoticize our research subjects by turning them into the Other. This process of Othering constructs, produces, and maintains difference, and there is always hierarchy involved in this difference. She echoes Rosaldo's assertion that while we may claim that all cultures are equal, anthropologists tend to see themselves as culturally invisible. Cultural visibility works along a steep gradient of inequality, in which those with less power tend to be seen as different and more culturally visible (Rosaldo 1993). As a partial corrective, Abu-Lughod suggests "writing against culture" by working against generalizations and a static notion of culture and writing instead about particular people, places, and events. Taking seriously the argument that "every view is a view from somewhere," anthropologists should dispense with the timeless present and offer a partial, situated view of real people caught up in the real events of their lives.

This book walks the line between generalities and particulars by focusing on stories of struggle, illness, and death in Saint Louis and Mumbaay, while illuminating wider process of communities caught up in economic crisis, livelihood shifts, and what I have come to think of as "the neoliberalization of just about everything." While the stories are rooted in the unique and contingent histories of the Saint Louis region, macrolevel processes of economic change and accompanying health sector reforms are unfolding throughout much of the developing world. My aim is to make people visible not for their cultural distinctness, but for the ways that their lives are intertwined with contemporary global processes of economic globalization and the transformation of health systems. By approaching these processes from the perspectives of people being affected by them, this book offers one slice of how these global trends articulate with the social hierarchies and cultural realities of a given place.

Critical Medical Anthropology (CMA) and the Practice of Health

As in the wider field of sociocultural anthropology, the main theoretical fault line in medical anthropology has been between interpretive orientations focused on the meaning and cultural construction of illness and suffering, and approaches based in political economy that emphasize the social production of disease and health inequalities. As medical anthropology coalesced into an identifiable subdiscipline in the post–World War II period, some of the earliest research focused on the therapeutic process and on understanding the social construction of health and healing in various societies (Csordas and Kleinman 1990; Janzen 1978; Kleinman 1980; Leslie 1976; Turner 1967). With the rise of Marxist approaches and critical theory in the 1970s, a critical school of anthropologists and sociologists integrated political economy into the emerging subfield (Doyal 1979; Frankenberg 1974; Morgan 1987; Morsy 1979, 1981; Singer 1986; Turshen 1984). These critical approaches sought to examine how global power relations, structural relations among economic systems, and political power shape the social field of health and patterns of disease (Morsy 1990).

The theoretical framework of critical medical anthropology was consolidated in the 1980s. Among other publications, the preeminent journal *Social Science and Medicine* published a special issue, "Towards a Critical Medical Anthropology" (Baer, Singer, and Johnsen 1986). CMA criticized "socioculturalism" for its narrow focus on symbol and ritual independent of political-economic context, for its failure to critique the power relations inherent in the healing encounter, and for failing to examine biomedicine's hegemony and relationship to capitalism (Singer 1989, 1193). In response to charges from the interpretive camp that the critical school was couched in narrow economic determinism (Gaines 1991), critical medical anthropologists acknowledged the importance of sufferer experience (Singer 1990) and sought to combine critical and interpretive concerns in their theory and ethnography (Baer 1997; Crandon-Malamud 1991; Farmer 1993; Lock and Scheper-Hughes 1987, 1990).

CMA is now a mainstream approach in medical anthropology, and the past two decades have seen sustained attention to how structural inequalities shape vulnerability to disease and access to medical care (Farmer 1993, 1997, 2004, 2005; Nguyen and Peschard 2003; Scheper-Hughes 1993). The rise of neoliberalism globally, the devastating effects of structural adjustment programs on health systems in developing countries, and the hegemony of market-based strategies in global health policy have made it all but impossible for medical anthropologists to ignore global political economy in their work. This book builds on research that has grappled with the ways that neoliberal economic policies have intersected with the social and political arena of health care delivery, health seeking, and vulnerability to disease (Castro and Singer 2004; Fort, Mercer, and Gish 2004; Hong 2004; Janes et al. 2006; Kim et al. 2000; Schoepf et al. 2000; Turshen 1999). Several of the tenets of CMA have shaped my approach: the claim that health is profoundly political; the assumption that class, race, and gender inequalities determine the distribution of health, disease, and health care; and the conviction that we must avoid an artificial separation of local settings and wider macroeconomic and political contexts (Castro and Singer 2004, xiv). My research aims to support the assertion that one of the important contributions of CMA can be "to provide insight about how health care systems work when subject to the exigencies of local power" (Pfeiffer and Nichter 2008, 412).

Beyond using critical medical anthropology as a theoretical point of departure, my research has also been influenced by the notion that practice theory helps us move beyond the impasse between critical and interpretive approaches in anthropology (Ortner 1984, 2006). While practice theory has shifted some of the central concerns of anthropology as a whole, medical anthropologists have found it particularly useful for posing questions about health, illness, and health action in the face of structural inequalities and constraints on making use of health-enabling resources. Building on Bourdieu to address the central concerns of health and illness, anthropologists have recognized health as another serious game that does not take place on a level playing field (Whiteford and Manderson 2000). The game of health is highly stratified depending on individual and family access to and embodiment of different forms of capital (Meinert 2004, 12). As such, health practice is part of one's habitus, and health action is "not a matter of lack of knowledge or irrational choice, but should be understood as the interplay of locally defined resources and competence to mobilize them" (Meinert 2004, 13).

A concern with health practice, meaning what people actually do when faced with affliction, illness, or vulnerability to mishap and misfortune, lies squarely at the center of this book. The study of health practice addresses how people experience, interpret, and respond to illness and attempt to mitigate the aspects of daily life that are thought to be problematic for health (Obrist 2003). I employ the notion of health practice to refer to an even larger domain of activity that encompasses government financing and organizing of health systems, medical district personnel carrying out the everyday tasks of running health facilities, neighborhood health committees vying for power over health funds, and the activities of men, women, and children who are trying to cope with illness. Using this broad concept of health practice, the book aims to capture the multiplicity of fields of health action, and to locate some of the dysfunction of the health system by pointing out the ways that social actors occupying different domains of health action misread or ignore the stakes and constraints of individuals in other fields.

Some kinds of health practice that become visible in this book are the daily actions of rural and urban families responding to numerous, overlapping afflictions. Families in Ganjool are caught in the grip of rural economic collapse, while shantytown dwellers in Pikine face a daily barrage of challenges from finding clean water to disposing of household waste. Employees of the Saint Louis medical district are charged with implementing government-backed reforms that may have little logic, relevance, or application in their particular context. Against the backdrop of these larger difficulties are the dozens of moments of daily jousting (and subsequent injuries) along the fault lines of gender, age, and generation that form the architecture of highly stratified Wolof society (Diop 1981, 1985). Through narratives of family illness, village development politics, and the tensions between neighborhood health committees and clinic nurses, we see how the local moral worlds of the household, village, neighborhood, and medical district are infused with the micropolitics of social relations and embedded within larger political economies. These local moral worlds provide contexts of shared history and experience that mediate larger social forces and shape their specific local effects (Kleinman 1986, 1992).

Methods

This book is based on twenty months of field research in Senegal between 1996 and 1999, with follow-up visits in 2002, 2005, and 2006. The study was conceived as a multi-sited ethnography (Marcus 1995); data were collected using a multi-site, multi-method approach, including focus groups, semi-structured interviews, participant observation, and a census of health resources in Pikine and Ganjool. I worked in several field sites because I wanted to document Senegal's experience with health sector reform from multiple perspectives. I hoped to capture the experiences of people on both sides of health care reform, that is, the Ministry of Health administrators and medical personnel, and the patients and community members who encountered these reforms when they pursued treatment at public dispensaries and hospitals. I sought the perspectives of the clinical personnel who were on the front lines of implementing changes to the formal health system, and the perspectives of people who were struggling to resolve health problems. The research design allowed me to explore a variety of views and experiences and to compare the outcome of health reform in urban and rural settings.

One focus of my study was the Senegalese Ministry of Health, including administration at the national level, administrators and health personnel at the district level, and medical staff working at neighborhood dispensaries and maternal child health centers. The primary geographic unit of analysis was the Saint Louis medical district, one of forty-five such districts in Senegal. The other two sites were the neighborhood of Pikine, the most socially, politically, and economically disadvantaged neighborhood in Saint Louis, and the rural community of Mumbaay in the Ganjool region in the Senegal River delta. The research was conducted in several phases, and each phase corresponded with a home base at one of the field sites.

I lived in Saint Louis for a period of eight months and I worked to become part of the community of health care personnel and administrators in the district by becoming a frequent visitor at their medical offices. Eventually I was invited to attend the monthly district staff meetings. These meetings proved to be the most important source of information on the organization of the district, the problems facing the medical personnel, and the conflicts between the personnel and the neighborhood health committees. Once I became a regular fixture at district meetings I was able to conduct interviews with administrative personnel and medical staff. In addition, I observed neighborhood health committee elections, and attended the district training sessions for the newly elected health committee officers. I made occasional visits to five of the district clinics and had informal conversations with staff during those times. To complement the perspectives of the medical personnel, I conducted interviews with health committee members from the Pikine and Get-Ndar health posts.

Working in the neighborhood of Pikine presented a host of challenges. In the wake of disastrous flooding in the summer of 1998 that forced many Pikine residents from their homes, I was not able to find housing there. Since I was living in another part of Saint Louis, the main difficulty was forging relationships with people through daily visits. As Pikine presented an unsolvable dilemma for sampling (a population of 45,000 and very little existing demographic information), I relied upon women's groups as my primary sources of data on neighborhood health issues and women's health practices. I became an honorary member of the only women's group in Pikine working on health issues, Xaal Yoon Wi, by attending their monthly group meetings and the tea-drinking parties held by the Xaal Yoon Wi community health workers. I spent nearly six months with the group before conducting interviews and focus groups with their members; this investment of time and our resulting camaraderie produced the richest and most candid data that I obtained in Pikine. I conducted focus groups with seven additional women's groups, and this data was supplemented by interviews with group members and participant observation in the three Pikine households where I spent most of my leisure time.

When I moved to Ganjool I arranged to have a room and a private bathroom added on to the home of my adopted aunt, and my close proximity to a number of family compounds gave me tremendous access to the inner workings of rural households. One of my early research activities was to map the village and all of its households, and I received much input from neighbors and friends as I worked on this map during teatime following the midday meal. My objective was to survey each of the households on the map to obtain basic demographic data on the village. While this was a complicated project that took weeks to complete, I succeeded by enlisting the help of the young woman in my household and the two community health workers. With the help of many Ngeyeen residents (my neighborhood in the village, so designated because of the prevalence of families with the surname Gey), I compiled a list of village medical resources, that is, individuals in the village with expert knowledge regarding the treatment of particular illnesses.

I frequently visited the health hut and had numerous conversations with the two health workers, and I accompanied ailing Ngeyeen residents on their visits to local healers and to the Tassinère health post to see the nurse. I also used more formal methodologies, such as illness interviews with male and female residents of Mumbaay. An informal focus group evolved among the women with whom I drank tea every evening after dinner. This group included one of the health hut workers and three other women who had married into the same household. The five of us gathered nearly every evening to reflect on the day's events, to listen to news on the radio, and to drink tea. These women were my closest friends and they were responsible for much of my insight into women's lives in the village.

Most of my free time every day was spent doing rounds and checking in with friends and acquaintances, most often in the immediate neighborhood of Ngeyeen. I visited people who were sick, and participated in local discussions about the malaria epidemic and other health problems. I attended many local ceremonies and social events such as weddings, baptisms, and funerals, and I helped with the onion harvest. I became accustomed to the rhythm of daily life in the village, and experienced disruptions to this rhythm during the two-month flood that prevented travel by car to Saint Louis, and during the malaria outbreak when nearly 75 percent of village members were gravely ill. Most of my socializing time was spent with the women who were my immediate neighbors, although the male members of my household provided some access to the world of men. They would report on the events and topics of discussion at the *grand place*, the spot at the center of the village where men of all ages gathered daily to socialize for several hours in the late morning and again before the late afternoon prayer.

The quality of my data on Mumbaay reflects the degree to which I was integrated into social networks as a household member, an in-law, a neighbor, and as a source of pharmaceuticals and occasional medical advice. To some I was a nuisance; to many I was a source of great entertainment. Generally, formal methodologies are very important for social scientists, but on the whole I achieved a greater understanding of women's lives and experiences through more informal means. While my Pikine data rely heavily on how women describe their lives, in Mumbaay I had the advantage of witnessing important events firsthand and participating in the discussions and debates about the meaning of these events.

The Production of Anthropological Knowledge

When students ask Kath Weston if she could have done her study of gay and lesbian kinship if she were not a lesbian, she replies, "No doubt, then again it wouldn't have been the same study" (Weston 1991, 13). Could this study have been done if I were not binational, fluent in Wolof, and married to a Senegalese man among whose family I collected much of my data? Undoubtedly, another anthropologist could have done this study, yet my access to people and the kinds of information they were willing to share (or conceal) was certainly shaped by my family connections. Feminist anthropologists have lobbied for social scientists to present themselves as real, historical individuals with situated perspectives, and to reflect critically on their social position and power relations within the communities they study (Abu-Lughod 1993; Harding 1991). The following is a brief sketch of some of the ramifications of my identity and social position on the research process.

Several things made it difficult for people to categorize me with the criteria normally used to label foreigners in Senegal. My language skills in Wolof immediately set me apart from the French nationals, who are often thought to be arrogant and hostile to local culture and national languages. The next assumption was that I must be a Peace Corps volunteer; they are well known and well liked because they usually learn a national language during their stay. However, because of their predominantly rural experience, Peace Corps volunteers are also seen as being unkempt or even dirty, rough around the edges, and culturally inappropriate when they come to the city. This prototype did not fit with my professional behavior and style of dress. As I was not French, not a Peace Corps worker, and not a development worker, I was outside of many people's frame of reference. In daily interactions many people assumed that I was born and raised in Senegal. While my language skills almost always guaranteed an instant in, they were also a handicap as people often assumed that I knew things that I in fact did not know.

As being Wolof is nearly synonymous with being Muslim, it was inconceivable to many people that I had not converted to Islam. Being married to a Muslim made my nonconversion even more difficult to understand. Although it was often uncomfortable to field questions about my religious status, it was evident that some people were truly concerned about my moral safety and well-being. One nurse's aide kept encouraging me to come to her house so she could teach me how to pray. During my only serious illness I was in Dakar and slept in my mother-in-law's bed, where she spent much of the night watching over me. After one of my numerous trips to the bathroom with dysentery, she had me recite prayers with her, assuring me that this was the best thing to do in a crisis. This gesture could be seen as subtle encouragement to convert, but it was also the most potent remedy she knew for illness. She had previously shared stories with me about some of the more difficult times in her life and how her faith enabled her to survive.

The extent to which having a Senegalese husband opened doors or altered my relationships with people varied in different contexts. In the most formal situations, such as seeking research clearance at the Ministry of Health, being able to introduce myself as "Madame Joob," and exchanging greetings in Wolof immediately placed me in a category that was one step closer to being Senegalese. While fluency in Wolof and my married name helped establish rapport in many formal and public situations, it was in the village that my access to people and information was most profoundly shaped by my marriage. My father-in-law was one of the more successful migrants from Ganjool to Saint Louis and one of the first from the village of Mumbaay. On more than one occasion I was told that if he were still alive things would be better in the village. His two surviving wives spent most of his modest fortune in the years immediately following his death. Consequently, the remaining family in Mumbaay is not part of the economic or political elite. Nonetheless, he established an enviable legacy in which seven of his fourteen children have permanently migrated to Europe or the United States.

The most explicit illustration of the importance of family ties occurred during my demographic survey in Mumbaay. Several people told me that it was only because I was their in-law that they were giving me information. Initially I brushed these comments off as playful banter, but later I learned that many village residents had refused to cooperate with enumerators sent by a local NGO to gather socioeconomic data for their child-sponsorship program. It seems that some village residents felt they couldn't refuse to help me because I was a legitimate village member with social leverage stemming from my family ties. Although I always attempted to gain consent before interviews and to respect people's privacy and confidentiality, it remains unclear whether village residents felt their cooperation with my study was entirely voluntary.

On the other hand, most villagers were very interested in my research and they were concerned that I not overlook them. When I started the household census in my immediate neighborhood, residents in other parts of the village reminded me that I hadn't been to see them yet. People also wanted to know about the results of my research. Was there money involved? Would I be bringing a development project? What was in it for them? These were difficult questions to answer, though I always emphasized that first and foremost I was doing research to complete my degree. At one point I acted as a liaison between the village and Plan International, but it is difficult to argue that Mumbaay residents gained anything from my research.

I often struggled to remain an anthropologist when other relationships with people threatened to overtake my commitment to conducting research. How could I view a friend as a source of data, or take field notes on family conflict that I was witnessing only because I was a family member? I faced having to turn friends and family members into informants, and I sometimes felt that to write ethnographically about people I knew and their lives was somehow to dehumanize them. There have been many critiques of anthropology's tendency to exoticize or to participate in radical othering and I often struggled with my own participation in this project. I have attempted to portray the individuals who appear in the book in all of their complexity so that they don't appear to be one-dimensional, and I have also attempted to render their experiences more familiar than foreign. I hope that I have adequately conveyed the nuances of daily life, and that by including people's own voices, thoughts, stories, and fears I have closed part of the gap between us and them.

As a final thought, I likely would not have chosen to conduct field research in Pikine or in Ganjool without these family connections. One of the greatest determinants of my position and social standing was my spouse, who had definite expectations about how I should behave and accommodate to village life. He played a very large role in image management, and he constantly reminded me about appropriate and inappropriate behavior, social obligations, and so forth. I faced continual warnings that certain subjects and approaches to data gathering were off limits. An important Wolof social value referred to as *sutuura* translates as privacy or discretion. I often had to forgo professional curiosity and my willingness to transgress some social norms in response to his strict warnings that I respect people's privacy.

Negotiating relationships of wife, in-law, neighbor, friend, village resident, and anthropologist proved complex, and I often longed for what I imagined to be the routine social relationships of other anthropologists who had a clear notion of their professional boundaries. Because I had access to information as a family member and not as an anthropologist, I have been very selective in choosing incidents and anecdotes to relate, and I have not recounted any stories about my in-laws' main household in Dakar. I have also protected people's identities by not using real names; unless otherwise indicated, all of the names found here are pseudonyms. In spite of my increased access to some aspects of life in Senegal, this study is still an outsider account.

Organization of the Book

Chapters 2 and 3 provide an overview of Senegal's colonial and postcolonial history and introduce the communities where this study took place. These chapters situate the current economic challenges facing the region within a historical context of marginalization and deeply rooted social inequalities. Though Saint Louis was once the bustling capital of French West Africa, since Senegal's independence in 1960 it has experienced political and economic decline coupled with booming population growth due to rural flight. Pikine, a shantytown neighborhood on the outskirts of Saint Louis, illustrates the countless problems that plague rapidly developing, unplanned peripheral neighborhoods in urban centers. The Ganjool region, located in the delta of the Senegal River, has been suffering agricultural decline since the opening of the Diama dam in 1988. Faced with a collapsing rural economy, the majority of Ganjool's young men have fled the region to work as migrant fisherman in Dakar or the Gambia. Instead of being caught up in the frenzy of economic growth and rapid global integration, these urban and rural communities represent the spaces suffering from ongoing decline. These chapters insist on bearing witness to the small tragedies unfolding in places like Pikine and Ganjool as they are part of the larger story of neoliberalism and globalization.

In chapter 4 I argue that the major turning point in global public health has been the implementation of market-based health reforms, which signaled the end of the commitment to "health for all" made by governments at the Alma Ata meetings in 1978. In this chapter I explain how these reforms instigated major restructuring of Senegal's health system, and signaled the exit of the state from social services. Though these reforms have often been referred to as "the new partnership" between the Senegalese government and its citizens, in actuality citizens have been all but abandoned with few resources to mitigate their vulnerability to disease. I examine the three main pillars of health reform in Senegal—privatization, decentralization, and participatory management structures—and describe the kinds of conflicts and tensions that have been associated with these reforms.

Chapter 5 provides an up-close look at the process of health sector reform from the perspectives of individuals living and working in Pikine. The case study of the collapse and gradual recovery of the Pikine health post demonstrates how health reforms often can't accomplish their stated objectives because of the ways in which they intersect with local social and political realities. Pikine's experience reflects some of the larger structural problems in the medical district, where health reforms have often worked to reinforce the power base of local elites while rendering medical care even less accessible to the urban poor. In the chapter I examine how the quality of medical care at neighborhood health posts in Saint Louis has deteriorated as a result of conflicts between medical personnel and local communities.

In chapter 6 I explore contested medical hegemonies and local health practices. I describe how health strategies reflect people's ability to mobilize preventative and curative therapies rooted in biomedicine, Islam, and Wolof medicine. In spite of biomedicine's global dominance in public health, biomedical diagnoses and "rational" biomedical behavior cannot simply replace existing ways of understanding and coping with illness. Instead, cultural frameworks for interpreting and responding to sickness operate as cultural filters for new information. Although men and women expend a tremendous amount of energy responding to sickness and maintaining health, their health actions remain largely invisible to medical professionals because they often rely on Islamic therapies and other local medical traditions. By examining the complexity of health practice, the chapter counters assertions of policymakers and medical professionals that ignorance and lack of formal education are the most significant obstacles to ameliorating health status in Senegal.

Chapters 7 and 8 provide an ethnographic account of contending with illness in Ganjool. In chapter 7 I explore the gendered power relationships within families and households to show how social and economic inequalities influence women's health practice. Using the stories of three wives and mothers, I demonstrate how household position affects women's ability to mobilize health resources. While polygyny creates certain dilemmas for Wolof women, having access to other adult women's labor buffers them from social and economic vulnerability. Understanding the constraints on women's health practice illuminates the tremendous discrepancy between the lived realities of sickness and death, and the idealized models of health participation and empowerment circulating in state discourses about health.

In chapter 8 I examine how the changing political economy of the Ganjool region articulates with highly stratified relations across generation. Building on chapter 7, this chapter provides a detailed analysis of family decision making in the face of grave illness. The chapter recounts three serious illness episodes, each involving young men whose medical care created conflict and disagreement among household members. Controlling young men's labor and movement has become increasingly challenging for senior men in Ganjool, and controlling the therapeutic process is one important way that heads of household can assert their remaining power. These cases illustrate how generational hierarchies mediate individual experiences of sickness, heighten vulnerability, and lead to neglect.

In chapter 9 I assess recent attempts to bring health development to Mumbaay in the form of new infrastructure, information, and the promotion of different kinds of health behavior. These development efforts attempted to transform local health practices by promoting new health resources and then motivating people to make use of them. They ultimately failed because they overlooked the ways that health strategies reflect cultural orientations to disease, and how power relations influence therapeutic decision making and access to health-enabling resources.

In my conclusion I assert that the contentious process of health reform in Senegal illuminates the global trends affecting people's lives in communities throughout sub-Saharan Africa. An ethnographic analysis of these macrolevel forces, and how they intersect with existing social, political, and economic realities, can deepen our understanding of contemporary health challenges in the context of neoliberal globalization. While recent critical literature in medical anthropology has emphasized structural violence as an important explanatory framework, in this chapter I emphasize the importance of engaging with both vertical and horizontal power relations operating in local communities and their influence on health practice and vulnerability to disease.

2

A Brief History of Senegal

This chapter offers an overview of Senegal's past and examines its seeming inability to overcome its present economic and political dilemmas. Over the course of its history, Senegalese society has been marked by profound social inequalities that have deep roots in the precolonial social order, the colonial experience, and the rise of political and religious elites before and after independence. Social inequalities were institutionalized in the precolonial era in aristocratic societies that were highly stratified by social order and caste. The era of French conquest and occupation, which coincided with the rise of dynamic Sufi organizations and a near-complete Islamization of the population, further entrenched disparities along lines of education, race, religion, language, and rural versus urban residence.[1] A small urban African elite obtained positions of power in the colonial administration, and Muslim leaders offered an imposing counterforce to French rule. Yet the vast majority was subject to French authority as colonial subjects, and willingly submitted to the moral authority of Sufi leaders as faithful disciples.

At independence, the nascent African political elite (urban, cosmopolitan, often educated in France) inherited the state apparatus and proposed a vision of modernity anchored in African socialism. But this ambitious rhetoric masked the vulnerability of state stability based on distributing wealth, jobs, and other resources in exchange for party loyalty. The implementation of structural adjustment programs in the 1980s and 1990s brought an end to decades of ineffective economic policy and highly centralized government control, yet the short and long-term returns on economic austerity have proved elusive. Decentralization has opened up new political spaces for contesting the ruling party's monopoly on state power, but for most Senegalese their dire economic opportunities overshadow any enthusiasm about an increasingly transparent and permeable state. Senegal's economic stagnation continues, and many

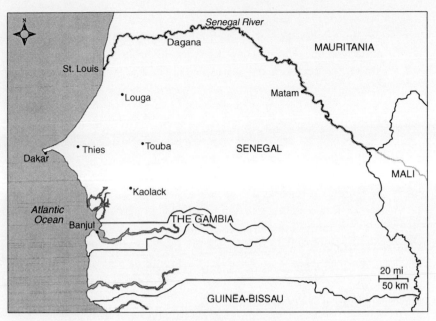

FIGURE 2.1 Map of Senegal

scholars point to the ruling classes' lack of political leadership and vision in the face of hegemonic neoliberalism. The question posed early in the days of structural adjustment remains: "Can Senegal emerge from the crisis?" (Duruflé 1994).[2]

Early History, Islam, and the Dawn of Colonization (1659–1854)

The precolonial social and political order of Senegal was characterized by the Wolof kingdoms (the majority ethnic group in Senegal) as well as the Sereer state and Fulbe kingdoms in the Fuuta Toro region of the Senegal River valley (Barry 1985; Diouf 1990; Gamble 1957). The largest precolonial monarchy, the Jolof empire, reached its peak in the mid-fifteenth century and then disintegrated when its constituent polities (the Wolof kingdoms of Baol, Cayor, Waalo, and the Serer states of Sine and Saluum) asserted their independence in the following century (Boulegue 1987). Precolonial Wolof and Fulbe society was stratified by social categories that many scholars have referred to as castes. These divisions included freemen, servile artisan castes (jewelers, blacksmiths, weavers, leather-workers, griots) and slaves (Diop 1981; Gellar 1982). The category of freemen included ruling lineages of the main Wolof states as well as peasants. Although of extremely low social status, domestic slaves sometimes owned land and married, and they were affiliated with specific families and could not be bought and sold, unlike trade slaves. Trade between the

Senegambia region and Europe dates from the fifteenth century; during the slave trade Senegal was the largest supplier of slaves until the end of the six-teenth century, when the trade moved farther down the Atlantic coast (Barry 1997; Curtin 1972). Clientelism or patron-client relationships were an important feature of the aristocratic monarchies; these relationships created social ties between rulers, nobles, and their dependents based on tribute and loyalty in exchange for protection (Gellar 2005). These social castes were indexed in part by family names, and though in contemporary Senegal many casted people have become wealthy entrepreneurs, successful politicians, or well-known scholars, caste status still carries a certain degree of stigma. Endogamous marriage within these social groupings remains the norm.

The early arrival of Portuguese explorers in the fifteenth century marked the first contact with Europeans, but the region had long been integrated into trans-Saharan trading circuits. Portuguese accounts from the fifteenth century report that Islam was followed by Wolof rulers and their entourages, but was only super-ficially observed by the general population (Babou 2007). For several centuries, Senegal's precolonial aristocracy participated in Sahelian and trans-Atlantic trade, and the regional political economy was heavily influenced by both, hence the argu-ment that Senegal has long been a nation "between Islam and the West" (Gellar 1982). The social and political turbulence of the centuries preceding French con-quest formed the backdrop against which the Wolof aristocracy increasingly lost power and legitimacy to Muslim leaders. With political shifts of the seventeenth and eighteenth centuries, Islam increasingly became "a refuge for the powerless, who were the primary victims of the violence and insecurity spurred by the slave trade, dynastic wars, and French encroachment" (Babou 2007, 31).

The emergence of locally based Sufi movements in the late nineteenth and early twentieth centuries, organized around the legacies and teachings of North African saints (the Qadiriyya and the Tijaniyya) and native sons, Amadu Bamba (the Muridiyya) and Abdoulaye Niasse (Niasse branch of the Tijaniyaa), set the stage for the reorganization of Wolof society in the wake of the slave trade and in the midst of French conquest. By the end of the nineteenth century Islam was widespread throughout the Senegambia region, and Muslim leaders seemed poised to reign over a new social order in Senegal. The Sufi orders (*tariqa*) were no match for France's expansionist impulse; France's military strength and commercial foothold in the region allowed it to "steal victory from the Islamic revolutionaries" in the mid-nineteenth century (Boone 2003, 49).

Saint Louis as a Base for Commerce and Conquest

The Compagnie du Cap Vert founded what would become the city of Saint Louis by building a trading post on the island in 1659; the Compagnie specialized in the trade in gum Arabic and slaves (Bonnardel 1992). The island of Saint Louis was a less than ideal site for the colonial fort and trading post, primarily because of its lack of freshwater and vegetation, the difficulty of disposing of waste, and the geographic limits to population growth. In spite of these challenges, Saint Louis became the base of French operations in West Africa; it served as the headquarters from which the French explored and eventually colonized the rest of Senegal, southern Mauritania, and Mali. Saint Louis was also the center of French commercial interests. Other Bordelais firms joined the Compagnie du Cap Vert and eventually came to dominate trade in the Senegalo-Mauritanian region. By the end of the eighteenth century, Saint Louis had a population of six thousand people, six hundred of whom were Europeans (Crowder 1967). The city reached the height of its colonial glory in the late nineteenth century, becoming the capital of French West Africa in 1895.

The city was built on an island at the mouth of the Senegal River approximately 2.5 kilometers long and 300 meters wide. The island was split into two halves, Nord and Sud (North and South, called Lodo and Sindone by the indigenous population), with military and commercial interests occupying the north and churches and residential areas occupying the south. The location of public infrastructure reflects the pattern of French occupation; even today the city's hospital, court, mayor's office, central police station, governor's mansion and administrative offices are all located on the island. During Faidherbe's tenure as Governor General (1854–1861 and 1863–1865) the city expanded beyond the borders of the island, first to the Langue de Barbarie, the strip of land west of the island along the Atlantic Ocean and then to the mainland. The Pont Servatius was inaugurated in 1856, connecting the island to the new neighborhoods of Get-Ndar, Ndar-Tuut, and Goxumbaaj along the ocean. The Ndar-Tuut market (which still flourishes today) was built in 1880, and many administrative offices for both Senegal and Mauritania were established along the main thoroughfare, Avenue Dodds (Ndiaye 1987). The mainland, referred to as Sor, was slow to be populated but experienced rapid growth after ferry service began from the island in 1858. The Pont Faidherbe, perhaps the most iconic symbol of the city, connects the island to Sor and was inaugurated in 1897 (Ndiaye 1987).

Early residents of Saint Louis included French military and merchants, particularly from Bordeaux, and the growing center of trade attracted refugees from the interior of Senegalo-Mauritania (Robinson 2000). Merchants often cohabitated with Senegalese women, a tradition that came to be known as *mariage à la mode du pays*. These unions often produced heirs that were recognized by their French fathers, bore their last names, and inherited their property, giving rise to the distinct *métis* (Creole) population on the island. The descendants of these unions were among the first Senegalese to receive a French education and to benefit from republican institutions that the French established in Saint Louis.

The French faced many challenges to keeping their military officers alive and healthy. The earliest medical facilities, such as the military hospital built

in 1819, served only the French population of Saint Louis. Military doctors staffed
the hospital, assisted by Catholic sisters who served as medical aides. In 1876
and 1888 dispensaries for the local population were built in Get Ndar and Sor
and run by Catholic sisters. The military phase of colonial biomedicine ended in
1897 when the military hospital became a colonial hospital; limited medical
facilities became available to the indigenous population in 1905 with the creation of the Assistance Médicale Indigène (Ngalamulume 1996).

Daily life in the fort was characterized by instability and fear of death and disease for the European population. The climate posed some problems, but the
greatest health risks were the lack of potable water and problems with waste,
which was dumped at the riverbanks and then in the middle of the river.
Residents bathed with river water and had poor diets that consisted largely
of meat, bread, and alcohol, with little fresh produce (Bonnardel 1992, 53).
Malaria and yellow fever were the main disease threats; during the eighteenth
and nineteenth centuries every yellow fever epidemic killed a third to one half of
the European population in just a few weeks (Bonnardel 1992, 54; Ngalamulume
1996).

Early European medical theories centered around environmental and sociocultural sources of disease; stagnant water, the hot/rainy season, and evil
winds were thought to cause illness, as did the sanitation habits and other
behaviors of the indigenous population (Ngalamulume 1996). The French
administration acted accordingly and passed public health decrees to clear the
center of the island of huts (starting in 1857), to create public toilets and sanitation inspectors (1882), and to ban the drying of fish and animal skins on the
island during the rainy season (1878, 1885). Other public health strategies
included fumigating houses, painting houses with lime, and creating health
inspections for all ships entering and leaving the colony. At the turn of the century, when it was known that mosquitoes were an important vector for malaria
and other illnesses, efforts were made to remove stagnant water and other
breeding grounds on the island (Ngalamulume 1996).

Prior to the germ theory of disease there was a limited understanding of
how yellow fever was transmitted, and local remedies included bloodletting and
the application of leeches. The hospital was undoubtedly a miserable place that
most people would avoid when sick as they (perhaps rightly) feared it would
accelerate their deaths (Ngalamulume 1996). During epidemics, the French
administration sent troops to quarantine camps, but these measures had little
effect as they were always taken after the disease had spread. In 1885 an
immunization for yellow fever was created at the Institut Pasteur in Tunisia.
Unfortunately for the population of Saint Louis, just as colonial medicine was
to benefit from medical advances such as the germ theory, the French began to
shift their base of operations to Dakar. Saint Louis would never benefit from the
majority of improvements made in public health in the colony.

The Civilizing Mission (1854–1960)

The era of French colonialism in West Africa is perhaps best understood as "the military occupation and subjection of West Africans to an administration they did not want, and whose imposition they often resisted bitterly" (Crowder 1968, 4). The notion of the civilizing mission conveys the ideology that the French deployed as justification for their brutal conquest of the territory that would become Afrique Occidental Française (AOF). While Enlightenment philosophy suggested the potential universal equality of all men, it was the "sacred duty" of the French to civilize African populations and to usher them into modernity. In the words of one colonial official, "We do not intend to enslave, but to increase their well-being while improving our own" (Lebon, Minister of the Colonies, 1897, as cited in Crowder 1968, 71).

Although the French established trading forts on the islands of Saint Louis and Gorée and along the banks of the Senegal River, French conquest began in earnest after the appointment of Louis Faidherbe as governor general of the colonies. During his tenure (1854–1865), Faidherbe brought a third of contemporary Senegal under French control. He was sent to Senegal to confront the Moorish threat to French trade along the Senegal River, and he is credited with annexing the south bank of the Senegal and establishing the colonial capital in Saint Louis (Crowder 1968). Given the poor results of early agricultural experiments, Faidherbe decided against turning Senegal into a settler colony and instead he promoted the cultivation of groundnuts by local peasant farmers. The cultivation of peanuts began as early as the 1840s, and within several decades peanuts were the foundation of the colony's economy. The promotion of groundnuts as a cash crop for export offered a new economic niche to Sufi leaders and their followers; with an apparent abundance of land and labor at the disposal of Murid religious leaders, the French encouraged the expansion of peanut cultivation. The Murids migrated westward through central Senegal, bringing new lands under cultivation (establishing the Groundnut Basin) and capitalizing on the profitable groundnut trade.

The expansion of colonial infrastructure, in particular the Dakar–Saint Louis railroad which opened in 1885, increased the presence of the French administration in the interior and improved its ability to extract wealth through the peanut trade. Peanut exports began before colonial rule, but French investment in ports, roads, and the railroad ensured that it would become the backbone of the colonial economy. By the 1890s there was hope that Senegal might become a profitable agricultural colony (Galvan 2004). The center of the peanut trade eventually moved southward from Saint Louis to Kaolack, but as late as 1920 port traffic through Saint Louis numbered 100,000 tons annually (Camera 1968). By the end of the 1930s, two-thirds of the rural population was engaged in peanut farming (Gellar 1982, 13–14). Rather than

accumulating profits by increasing agricultural productivity, the French administration and French commercial houses extracted wealth from Senegal's peasants by commanding a monopoly on trade. The dominance of "merchant
capital" and the absence of capitalist investment in industry or improved technologies would prove to be an economic Achilles' heel for Senegal's economy
after independence (Boone 1992).

Senegal's modern political history has been marked by French experiments
with political, economic, and cultural assimilation. France's assimilationist policy
began before Faidherbe's tenure; after the French Revolution the Second Republic
decided to offer the colonies the power to send a representative to the French
National Assembly. In 1872 Gorée and Saint Louis achieved the status of full-
fledged French municipalities with the same rights as those in France; Rufisque
and Dakar were added in 1887. From this period onward a number of institutions
of civil society flourished in the colony and provided an arena within which different constituents could maneuver for power and influence. The most important
of these were electoral institutions created and maintained by the Third Republic
in the Four Communes; these included city councils, mayorships, a Senegalese
deputy in the French National Assembly, and a General Council with ten members
from Saint Louis and six from Rufisque (Johnson 1971; Robinson 2000).[3] The participation of residents of the Four Communes in colonial politics created a
vibrant political culture in which French merchants jockeyed for power with
Africans and métis. From the early establishment of local councils, municipalities, and finally the deputyship in the colony, the métis populations, *originaires*
(black Senegalese who had French citizenship) and the French competed for
influence and control of these political institutions (Babou 1997).

Though the métis notables initially dominated the electoral institutions—
particularly the rival Devès and Descemet clans—black Africans had increasing
access to French education and became effective political organizers by the turn
of the century (Babou 1997). The election of Blaise Diagne as the first black deputy
in 1914 (with a campaign financed partially by the Murids) signaled the end of the
métis dominance of local politics. The métis became advisers and supporters of
African politicians (Johnson 1971; Robinson 2000). Diagne played a crucial role in
recruiting African soldiers to assist France during the First World War, and he
used assimilationist discourse to try to increase the political rights of the originaires in the Four Communes and the French "subjects" living in the interior. This
eclipse of the métis paralleled Saint Louis' declining importance in the colony to
Dakar, the new regional and colonial capital. Dakar became the capital of the AOF
in 1902, but Saint Louis remained prominent as the joint capital of the colonies of
Senegal and Mauritania and as a center of trade and commerce.

The experiments with political, cultural, and economic assimilation were
embedded within the larger project of French colonialism, which was steeped in
certainty of France's moral, racial, and technological superiority. France's

assimilation strategies may have been based on a belief in the potential equality of all men, but the civilizing mission intended to use French influence and education to eliminate the cultural and racial differences between the French and their African subjects (Crowder 1967). The French administration did not extend this assimilationist policy beyond Senegal's Four Communes (and many colonial officials would come to regret the political rights that had been granted to residents of the Four Communes). Beyond the communes lay the colony, where Africans had the legal status of subjects and were ruled through administrative districts called circles and cantons headed by French commanders and French-selected African chiefs. Africans who were not citizens but subjects were forced to work for the administration, and taxation encouraged the growth of cash crops or selling labor. The chiefs were the much-despised agents of the colonial administration as they were charged with collecting taxes and recruiting men for labor gangs (Crowder 1968).

If a dynamic political culture emerged in the Four Communes, those in the countryside "lived under harsh rule with little identification with French culture or political systems" (Gellar 1982, 13). The emerging Sufi tariqa provided leadership and some refuge from colonial domination, and the French sought to suppress their influence. They exiled the charismatic leader of the Murids, Amadu Bamba, to Gabon and then to Mauritania, but with each exile his prestige and popularity grew. Eventually the French administration came to realize that Sufi leaders did not seek political authority over their followers, only spiritual authority and the right to preach and teach peacefully. From the early twentieth century, the French and the Muslim leaders embarked on a strategy of cooperation and accommodation to one another (Babou 2007; Robinson and Triaud 1997; Robinson 2000). The contemporary balance of power between the Senegalese state and Muslim leaders, each of which seeks to influence the population as citizens and disciples, respectively, has its roots in the patterns of accommodation established under French colonial rule (Villalon 1995).

Both of the world wars had a significant impact on French rule in Senegal. In the First World War, Blaise Diagne, Senegal's deputy to France, played a crucial role in recruiting West African troops (called *tirailleurs Sénégalais*) to fight for France. Although Diagne made a persuasive case that fighting for the *métropole* would bring greater enfranchisement to Africans living under French rule, the administration did not fulfill his promises to African soldiers (Crowder 1967). In the period following the war, twenty new representatives from the protectorate were added to the colony's General Council, which created a more visible power struggle between Senegalese with French citizenship (originaires) and French subjects. Crowder (1967) suggests that the political battles of the 1930s indicate the vast sociocultural distance between the originaires and French subjects.

During World War II, Africans in the AOF suffered under the Vichy regime, which revoked all of the political rights that had been granted to the residents of the Four Communes (Gellar 1982). At the Brazzaville conference in 1944, French general Charles de Gaulle proposed new reforms to promote social and economic development in the colonies. While these reforms were likely an attempt to counter a growing momentum for African independence, when they passed in 1946 they abolished forced labor, they ended the distinction between citizens and subjects, they extended suffrage and political representation to Africans living in the interior of Senegal, and they created a new Economic and Social Development Fund (Gellar 1982, 17). These trends toward increasing the social and political rights of Africans in the AOF furthered decentralization of the colonial administration and laid the groundwork for independence in 1960.

The emergent ruling class at independence descended from the urban elites who had enjoyed the rights of French citizenship for much of the colonial period. From almost the earliest phases of French presence in Saint Louis, Senegalese elites and the sons of prominent métis families were educated in France. While Crowder (1967) tends to emphasize the success of assimilation in the Four Communes, Senegalese historian Mamadou Diouf (1998) reminds us that the originaires may have been politically and economically French, but they were not culturally French. Diouf argues that the originaires formed their own cosmopolitan culture born of the processes by which "people possessed and exploited possibilities for hybridizing and selecting modes of acculturation" (Diouf 1998, 676). Regardless of the extent to which assimilation succeeded in fostering a rapprochement with French culture and values, in the course of their studies in the metropole Senegalese encountered "the deep streak of racism lurking just beneath the rhetoric of rights of man and universal culture" (Galvan 2004, 36). This experience of alienation, shared by both Africans and Afro-Caribbeans in France, gave rise in the 1930s to *négritude*, a social and cultural movement that romanticized and celebrated black culture in the face of a colonial impulse to efface it and deny its history.

Aimé Césaire and Léopold Sédar Senghor were young intellectuals from Martinique and Senegal, respectively, who had been educated in France and who served as the defiant voices of négritude. The concept of négritude laid claim to an authentically black civilization that countered the French notion of a universal European modernity to which colonized populations should aspire. As part of this trend toward Africanization, in the late 1930s many Senegalese political parties broke away from French parties as part of an effort to reclaim a unique set of values (evident in African history, culture, art, etc.) that could inform a new political philosophy. As an aspiring politician who would become independent Senegal's first president, Senghor advanced the idea of an "African socialism" based not in class struggle but in African values of communitarianism and reciprocity (Crowder 1967).

After the enfranchisement of Senegal's rural population with the elimination of the citizen/subject distinction in 1946, Senghor maneuvered to secure the support of the rural electorate in general, and the Murid *marabouts* (leaders) in particular (Boone 1992).[4] By 1948 Senghor founded a new political party in Senegal based on an anti-assimilation platform that called for recognizing African culture (Crowder 1967). His new party, dovetailing the French strategy of indirect rule, aimed to incorporate existing clientelistic networks into its sphere of support (Boone 1992). In 1951 Senghor's new party won both seats in the National Assembly, and he began to consolidate the political capital that would ensure his success at becoming independent Senegal's first president. These alliances revolved around a patronage form of politics in which rising power brokers rewarded supporters and those in their networks with political favors, state resources, employment opportunities, and so forth.

Independence and Beyond: From a Single-Party State to a Stable Democracy (1960–2000)

By the late 1950s the demand for African independence was being made by nationalist movements throughout the continent. While Anglophone leaders like Kwame Nkrumah and Julius Nyerere paved the way for independence in Ghana and Tanzania, Senegalese leaders were navigating France's latest political maneuver, the *loi cadre*. The law intended to stave off demands for independence by giving all of France's African territories democratic government with legislative power (Crowder 1967). The law generated debates about autonomy and a split from France, and in 1958 the first political party was formed in Senegal calling for independence. In the same year, De Gaulle formulated a new referendum for Franco-African relations and gave each colony three choices: integration into the French republic, self-government within a French commonwealth, or immediate independence (Gellar 2005, 43). Importantly, Senegal's Muslim leaders feared that an independent state would bring about a decline in their influence, and they came out strongly in favor of remaining within a French commonwealth. Senegal's political elite recognized the importance of strategic alliances with Sufi leaders, and the early pronouncement in favor of the commonwealth effectively leveraged similar support from the main political parties (Villalon 1995, 206). In spite of some lobbying for an independence vote in Senegal, all countries voted to remain with France except Guinea. The commonwealth proved to be short-lived as each of the colonies pursued a path to independence. The momentum for regional integration and autonomy nonetheless produced an attempt at a four-member federation of Senegal, Mali, Upper Volta, and Dahomey, but this quickly collapsed. Senegal and Mali tried to remain united in their own federation, which successfully declared independence from France in 1960. The federation of Mali quickly collapsed; within two months Senegal withdrew and successfully sought United Nations recognition as an independent country (Crowder 1967, 75–80).

Some scholars have attributed Senegal's postcolonial stability to its historical experience with democratic politics (Diouf 2001; Gellar 2005), while others stress the powerful Sufi orders as an effective counterbalance to hegemonic state power (Villalon 1995). Léopold Sédar Senghor, independent Senegal's first president, established political alliances with the rural elite and religious leaders in the 1950s that ensured the long reign of his party through his own tenure as president (1960–1980) and that of his successor, Abdou Diouf (1981–2000). Senghor's dominance of Senegalese postcolonial politics was not a foregone conclusion, as the period from 1960 to 1963 witnessed a fierce competition between Senghor and his rival party member Mamadou Dia. After Dia was found guilty of a coup d'état and sentenced to life in prison, Senghor presided over a one-party state in which his Union Progressive Sénégalais (UPS) party held all elected positions from 1963 to 1975 (Gellar 1982). Senghor shifted his strategy in the mid-1970s, first granting legal status to Adoulaye Wade's opposition party, the PDS (Social Democratic Party) in 1974 (the same year Dia was released from prison). Senegal's political field continued to widen, with constitutional amendments allowing three parties, then a fourth in 1979, and an unlimited multiparty system in 1981 (Gellar 1982).

One of the challenges for Senghor and his fellow party members, who inherited the colonial state, was Senegal's dire economic prospects. The French had been motivated more by expansion of empire than by economic gain, and there was very little investment in increasing Senegal's agricultural productivity or industrial base during the colonial period (Boone 1992; Crowder 1968). In the classic model that would be critiqued by dependency and world systems theorists in the 1960s and 1970s (Frank 1969; Rodney 1973; Wallerstein 1979), in the years following independence Senegal was heavily dependent on its ongoing relationship with France. Over 80 percent of Senegal's foreign trade was with France, the peanut harvest was sold to France at subsidized prices, France provided two-thirds of Senegal's foreign aid and almost all foreign technical assistance, French investors provided 90 percent of private capital and owned most industries, and France's treasury covered Senegal's foreign trade deficits (Gellar 1982, 51). After an early period of relative calm, the first economic crisis occurred in the late 1960s when successive droughts and stagnation in peanut production illuminated the state's economic vulnerability (Diop 2004).

Senghor took steps to reduce Senegal's dependence on France by selling peanuts on the world market, nationalizing the French military bases and sending most French troops home to France, and by requesting foreign aid from other countries (Crowder 1967). One of the major initiatives of the new government was to nationalize the peanut trade immediately after independence, which created alarm among Murid leaders who were concerned that they might lose their base of power (Boone 1992). Senghor also embarked on a series of national development plans that mobilized his notion of "African socialism." The state would take over large sectors of the economy, and *animation rurale* (community development) would be a primary focus of state investment. Senghor ultimately could not substantially reform the agricultural sector because his power base depended on alliances with the rural elite, who profited (along with the state) from extracting surplus from peasants. In spite of rhetoric about economic growth and animation rurale, Gellar concludes that the postindependence ruling elites did little to actually transform the state, but instead sought to reform it so that it would benefit national rather than metropolitan interests (1982). Senegal's postindependence political economy has been characterized by patron-client networks in which elites, rather than forming a capitalist class, instead accumulated wealth and status by access to the social capital and spoils of state power (Boone 2003).

In the 1970s Senegal, like much of the developing world, took on high levels of debt in the name of state-led national development. Senghor's development plans attempted to promote growth, economic diversification away from reliance on the peanut monoculture, and greater food sufficiency. During the colonial period the French had long dreamed of turning the Senegal River Valley into a bread basket for the region. The first dam to keep saltwater out of the river was built at Diama in 1947 in an attempt to promote irrigated agriculture in the Middle Valley of the Senegal River, and there were early attempts to promote industrial-scale rice and sugar production in the delta region near Saint Louis (Boone 2003). Senghor's government attempted to introduce cotton, sugar cane, and tomatoes in the Waalo region, and it created and financed small-scale rice irrigation projects. Senegal also joined together with Mali and Mauritania to create the Organisation pour la Mise en Valeur du Fleuve Sénégal (OMVS) to pursue a mega-infrastructure project involving dams in Manantali, Mali, and Diama, Senegal.

These ambitious projects gained momentum in the 1970s with the rise of peanut and phosphate prices (phosphates are one of Senegal's few exploitable natural resources), but by the late 1970s world prices dropped and Senegal was heavily in debt with acute needs for food imports and oil. The new irrigated perimeters in the Middle Valley "failed to produce enough rice to reduce dependency on imported rice, disrupted traditional production systems, and aggravated Senegal's foreign debt" (Gellar 2005, 50); meanwhile, the contentious collaboration of the OMVS also failed to produce the desired outputs of hydroelectric power or an agricultural revolution in the Senegal River Valley.[5] In the face of mounting international debt, after passing a stabilization plan (1978–1979), Senghor's prime minister Abdou Diouf (soon to be Senghor's successor as president) negotiated Senegal's first economic-recovery loan with the International Monetary Fund (IMF) in 1980, thus aligning Senegal's economic strategies with the recommendations of the Washington Consensus.

Although Senghor's African socialism did little to advance economic prosperity in the early independence period, his mastery of international diplomacy and reputation as Senegal's poet-president ensured a legacy of political and cultural prominence for Senegal. During his presidency arts and culture flourished in Senegal with the creation of the Ecoles Nationales Supérieur d'Arts plastiques and Ballet la Linguere, and the establishment of the Festival Mondial des Arts Nègres (Harney 2004). Senghor was a supporter of *la francophonie*, a loose commonwealth of former French territories, and he maintained a special relationship with France as a cornerstone of his foreign policy. A leading African intellectual, Senghor was the first African to be elected a member of the prestigious French Academy. He facilitated Senegal's rise to being one of the most active and influential African countries on the international scene by maintaining close links to France and brokering ties with Egypt, the PLO, and by making Senegal a member of the Islamic Conference (Gellar 1982, 67). Under Senghor, Senegal also became a major player in the "Group of 77," a coalition of developing countries seeking to redress economic and political inequalities between the developed and developing world. Senghor's presidency produced a number of paradoxes, including "a weakness of institutions and formal activities, an explosion of the informal sector, an extraordinary international reputation, fame of many Senegalese artists, a stable democracy, and a weak economy that required the constant pursuit of foreign aid" (Diouf 2001, 209).

While Senghor's diplomatic legacy might be enviable, Abdou Diouf inherited a highly centralized state on the verge of major economic crisis.[6] The near failure of the peanut crop in 1981 eliminated any hopes of avoiding an economic austerity lending package from the IMF, and Diouf had to shepherd the country through "its most politically and economically delicate phase since independence" (Diop 2002, 12). With the conditionalities of bailouts from the IMF came the neoliberal reforms that have become common throughout the world: deregulation, privatization of state industries, and liberalization of trade regulations. In spite of signing on to the austerity packages, Diouf and his administration "were not disciplined agents of the IMF and World Bank in the 1980s" (Diop 2004, 13). The government's ability to massage budgets and finesse economic indicators came to a conclusive end with a World Bank audit of public finances in 1993, marking a turning point in Senegal's relationship with the bank and the IMF. The government agreed to a *plan d'urgence* and liberalization began in earnest, but these late actions were not enough to avoid a 50 percent devaluation of the west African franc (CFA) in 1994 (Diop 2004).

To date their have been few positive outcomes from structural adjustment. By the end of the 1990s there were clear signs that poverty in Senegal had worsened, health infrastructure was deteriorating, children faced great difficulty attending school, and households were sacrificing spending on health and education to ensure their basic survival. The rise of neoliberalism in Senegal has also created a vacuum of political vision, leadership, and any political discourse alluding to social or political development; the ruling class has all but abandoned any pretense of state-led development (Diop 2004). As argued by Leys (1996), in the neoliberal era the only possible development strategy is not to have one; instead, national governments are charged with opening their borders to global capitalism and creating attractive enclaves for foreign investment. Perhaps most troubling to critics of neoliberalism is the rise of a new kind of global elite, the finance technocrats who now wield tremendous power over national economies and global economic relations (McMichael 1996). This new elite has not only risen to power, but has "escaped the ballot box and democratic checks and balances all the while proposing reforms that have a significant social and political impact" (Diop 2004, 14).

As in other parts of the world, calls to adopt liberal economic reforms in Senegal were accompanied by efforts to decentralize the national government. Senegal represents a particularly acute case of top-heavy and bloated state bureaucracy. The historical legacy of French bureaucracy weighs heavily in Senegal as evidenced by a high degree of centralization in government, the sheer size of government bureaucracy, the continued emphasis on procedural rules in the functioning of government, and the notion that "the task of applying these procedures is seen as the legitimate job of a bureaucratic elite trained especially in the technical skills of administration" (Villalon 1995, 80). Steps toward decentralization began in 1990 when urban mayors and the presidents of rural councils were given the right to create and manage local budgets; this was a significant shift as these budgets had previously been managed by state officials rather than local ones (Gellar 2005, 56). This process continued with Senegal's 1996 decentralization legislation that was designed to localize fiscal responsibility and decision-making, in part by creating regional councils in each of Senegal's ten regions.

The process of decentralization significantly changed Senegal's political landscape. With new arenas of power available in regional political contests, Senegal's opposition parties, which had been largely uncompetitive on the national political scene, began to participate in local politics. Nonetheless, the centralized state still controls the process of decentralization itself and rarely disburses enough funds to allow local government to carry out its new role effectively (Gellar 2005). Gellar's analysis echoes Villalon's observation that in the early 1990s local officials were often surprised by decentralization decrees being passed in Dakar, "that local state officials have frequently been caught off guard . . . indicates the degree to which even decisions about decentralization have been centralized in Senegal" (1995, 89). Other studies of decentralization suggest that they did not disrupt the fundamental power relations between party elites and the impoverished majority in rural and urban areas. Although decentralization is designed to increase the participation of stakeholders in local decision-making, Boone suggests that in the Peanut Basin the groundnut elite captured decentralized institutions and used this new access to local power to expand its control of local resources (Boone 2003).

Alternance and Beyond: Senegal in the Twenty-first century

Senegal's opposition parties long argued that Senegal would only be a proven democracy after the achievement of *alternance*, that is, regime change through the successful transfer of power from the ruling party to the opposition through democratic elections. In 2000, Abdoulaye Wade, who had been part of the opposition since the mid-1970s, finally achieved electoral victory and became Senegal's third president. Wade was supported by a wide coalition of urban and rural youth, intellectuals, trade unions, and large portions of the populace who had grown disenchanted with twenty years of Parti Socialiste (PS) rule. The 2000 elections brought a new wave of optimism to the Senegalese population that had been living for nearly twenty years under the grinding poverty and economic stagnation associated with structural adjustment. Perhaps the crowning moment in recent history was Senegal's victory over France in the 2002 World Cup. Beyond the symbolic value of defeating the former colonial power, after the match Senegalese citizens displayed a buoyant nationalism that revealed the depth of the population's desire to achieve a level of standing and belonging on the international stage.

Sadly, the population's hopes for alternance have proved largely unfounded. As Wade's Parti Démocratique Sénégalais (PDS) became the ruling party, "those in power continued to sing their own praises, favor their friends and clients, and work to use the system to make sure they would stay in power" (Gellar 2005, 89). Given the global hegemony of liberal economic policies, it is unsurprising that Wade has offered little vision for Senegal's economy beyond turning the capital city into a regional hub for capitalist expansion into West Africa. After successfully bidding to host the World Islamic Conference in 2007, Wade leveraged his religious and political ties to attract millions in Saudi and Kuwaiti investment in urban and rural development projects. What followed were several years of frenzied modernization and infrastructure projects in Dakar that came at great inconvenience to urbanites and at the expense of rural dwellers, who continue to be largely forgotten in the rush to build a cosmopolitan center of business for the region.

The state's commitment to liberalization, privatization, and decentralization continues, as groups that "formerly called themselves Senegalese patriots have dropped their revolutionary passions and have come to adhere to neoliberal principles" (Diop 2004, 16). In spite of this shift, Senegal's experience suggests the resilience of existing power relations and clan politics even in the face of externally driven efforts at reform. State power remains concentrated at the highest levels of government, and traditional power brokers have maintained their hold in spite of the changing terrain. Nonetheless, there have been some significant changes in the neoliberal period, particularly in the health sector. The adoption of cost recovery schemes in the health system (part of the Bamako Initiative package of reforms) marked a radical departure from the commitment since independence to provide the population with free medical care. The Senegalese experience with these globally driven health reforms is the subject of chapter 4.

Senegal's history has long demonstrated a unique balance between Islam and secular democracy, but the past decade has seen the rise of fundamentalist challenges to the secular state. Debates about revising Senegal's 1972 Family Code and the recent push for parity among men and women in elected office have spurred new demands for the restoration of Muslim courts and *sharia* law for Muslim families. Wade has been criticized for his personalization of presidential power and his flouting of legal and constitutional norms (Coulibaly 2003), yet he has proved himself to be a strong defender of Senegal's existence as a secular, democratic state (Gellar 2005, 164).[7]

Religious, cultural, and political debates in the public sphere can be quite heated, but Senegal's economic dilemmas continue to be at center stage in domestic and international media. Economic migration within sub-Saharan Africa and to Europe and North America has long been a favored strategy of Senegalese, and the Soninke and Murid diasporas have proven adept at establishing cohesive migrant communities abroad and fueling development projects and investment in their home regions. Yet one of the much-touted ironies of neoliberalism is the simultaneous drive to increase the mobility of global capital while attempting to stem the flow of labor. As the opportunities for legal migration dwindle, Senegalese youth have turned by the thousands to the possibility of clandestine passage to Europe via the Canary Islands in wooden fishing boats. Though the scores of fatalities have captured the world's attention, Senegal has found few solutions for its youngest generations. In an unusual move, the Spanish government has increased its development aid to Senegal in hopes that vocational training for young men will attenuate the push factors that cause so many to migrate illegally. In light of the desperation that has gripped Senegal's young people, it is difficult to be optimistic that such ad hoc efforts at economic development will offer a long-term solution.

Senegal's prospects in the near future appear modest at best. The reelection of Abdoulaye Wade in 2007 met with little enthusiasm at home or abroad, and he has produced little in the way of a coherent vision for Senegal's political or economic future. To be sure, Senegal continues to enjoy a stellar international reputation as a stable democracy, a cultural and artistic crossroads that produces international pop and film stars, and a moderate Islamic country aspiring to greater leadership in the Muslim world. Although it shares the historical legacy of the slave trade, European conquest, and recent independence with its West African neighbors, it is equally shaped by the remnants of precolonial social and political structures, the rise of Sufi orders, a singular experience with French assimilation, and the legacy of négritude and African socialism. While Senegal's future remains uncertain, regions like Saint Louis, which are peripheral to the state's political and economic ambitions, are in a doubly precarious position. The following chapter offers a closer look at Saint Louis' history and current challenges.

3

Urban and Rural Dilemmas

Much like the country as a whole, for the past several decades urban and rural residents of the Saint Louis region have confronted increasingly difficult economic conditions. While global capital and state development plans have skipped over this region, finding it unusable, many people have been left behind who are struggling to make do under worsening conditions (Ferguson 2006). They are caught between the empty promises of the state and various donors, and the neoliberal imperative for a privatized, downsized, decentralized government. Pikine residents have been waiting for neighborhood zoning since the early 1980s; meanwhile, the city government insists that it can't provide any additional services until Pikine becomes a regular neighborhood. The farmers of Ganjool were never informed about the environmental damage that the Diama dam would have on their agricultural lands and water supply. As the productivity of their soils decreases and their wells become increasingly salty, they face intense competition from farmers in the Middle Valley of the Senegal River who now grow red onions, Ganjool's main cash crop. Caught in these shifting political economies, Pikine and Ganjool represent two peripheries of a declining city and region.

Although Saint Louis carries an important legacy as one of the earliest sites of French settlement in West Africa and the former capital of Afrique Occidentale Française, it is now an aging historical landmark faced with dozens of problems common to African cities. After the transfer of the nation's capital from Saint Louis to Dakar in 1960, the city of Saint Louis slumbered in the wake of its more dynamic counterpart. With no industrial base to fuel local economic development, the city has been unable to maintain or expand its existing infrastructure. Walking among the crumbling colonial buildings downtown, it is easy to imagine that you are walking through a movie set dating from the early twentieth century. Some efforts to restore and preserve Saint Louis' colonial architecture are underway, so the city offers visitors a view of arrested decay juxtaposed with

37

new construction and the rubble of buildings too far gone to salvage. Insufficient infrastructure, shantytown neighborhoods on the borders of town, and a general lack of an economic pulse make the city feel like a sleepy backwater only partially buoyed by its illustrious past. The city is still the capital of the Saint Louis region, but the region as a whole has become largely marginal to Senegal's political scene and economic future.

Most of Saint Louis' recent demographic growth was spurred by the severe droughts of the 1970s and 1980s; thousands of peasants from the Senegal River Valley flocked to towns and cities to escape the escalating poverty in rural zones. By the mid-1980s several new neighborhoods had developed around Saint Louis's peripheries. Pikine, a shantytown on the southern outskirts of the city, is one of these chaotic products of rapid, unplanned urbanization. Although Saint Louis proper is now a tourist hub, Pikine residents live at the margins of town and typically lack access to urban amenities such as running water, electricity, basic sanitation services, public schools, and formal sector employment. Despite numerous failed attempts at *lotissement* (legal zoning), Pikine remains emblematic of the neglected neighborhoods in African cities that have experienced rapid urbanization.

While the city of Saint Louis began its decline shortly after Senegal's independence, the Ganjool region (located south of the city in the delta of the Senegal River) has experienced a much more recent crisis linked to shifts in state development priorities. In the 1970s an initiative emerged to promote food security and agricultural growth by developing the Senegal River Valley. Under the auspices of the Organisation pour la Mise en Valeur du Fleuve Sénégal (OMVS), the nations of Mali, Mauritania, and Senegal organized to harness the potential of the Senegal River. The focus of the project was to construct two large dams, one at Manantali in Mali and one just north of Saint Louis at Diama. At the Manantali dam, engineers can control the downriver flow of water, and the anti-salt dam at Diama ensures that the water above the dam remains fresh throughout the dry season. According to the logic of the project, eliminating seasonal salinization allows for the development of irrigated fields along the river, primarily intended for rice production. As a bonus to the agricultural projects, a hydroelectric power station at Manantali was to provide energy for the three countries.

Three decades and millions of dollars after the project was first conceptualized it has failed to achieve nearly all of its objectives. Irrigated agriculture has not resolved farmers' problems, and the artificial floods from Manantali that should have enabled farmers to continue floodplain agriculture have been irregular and ill-timed (Adams 2000; P. Dia 1998). The brief period of optimism for the economic rejuvenation of the region passed, leaving many farmers in the valley in worse condition than before. The failures of the project notwithstanding, the agricultural zone downstream from the Diama dam, including Ganjool, was

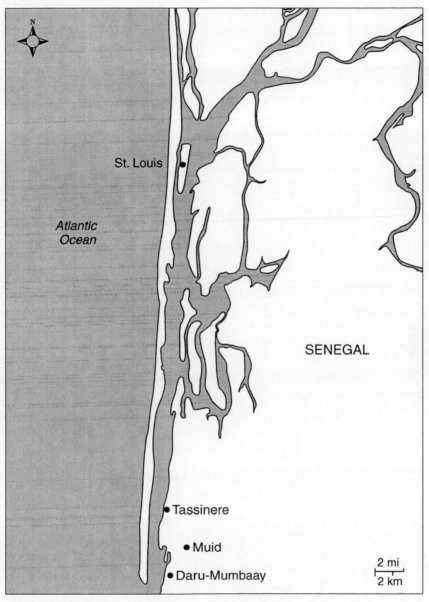

FIGURE 3.1 Map of St. Louis

Map by Tracy Ellen Smith

left out of the plan to improve agriculture along the river. From the earliest pro-jections of project results, Ganjool was included in calculations of environmen-tal degradation with no expected benefits to local residents from the dams and controlled flooding. Environmental impact assessments that predicted a rise in salt content of the water table and soils in the areas below Diama have proven accurate, and these negative effects are now being documented (A. Dia 1999). The latest plans for protecting this zone, which is "rich in biodiversity of both flora and fauna," propose stemming environmental damage in the hopes of pro-moting ecotourism, rather than protecting the livelihood of thousands of farmers there (UICN 1999). The Ministry of Environment has launched ecotourism ventures in Ganjool to promote environmental sustainability and income-generating activ-ities for local residents, a large portion of whom have already gone elsewhere to escape the region's economic stagnation.

Saint Louis: From Colonial Glory to "Dry City"

The city of Saint Louis still bears the prestige of being the first colonial city of l'Afrique Française Occidentale (AOF). The French built their city on a small island in the Senegal River that was previously only sparsely populated by Wolof fishing communities. Established first as a military fort and then as a comptoir, Saint Louis was the center of the gum trade and peanut exports in the nineteenth century as well as the headquarters for the French colonial administration and armed forces. Following the violent conquest of the interior of Senegal and Mauritania, trade flourished throughout the nineteenth and twentieth centuries. Saint Louis devel-oped into a busy administrative center that was the political and economic capital of the colonies. The administrative capital of the AOF was moved to Dakar in 1902, but Saint Louis remained the capital of Senegal and Mauritania, and it was the economic anchor for the region of the Middle Valley of the Senegal River and southern Mauritania. At independence in 1960, Mauritania built its own capital in Nouakchott, and the capital of Senegal was transferred to Dakar. This transfer marked the culmination of Dakar's economic and political growth and its eclipse of Saint Louis after the capital's transfer; the expatriate population, including the remaining commercial interests, vacated Saint Louis for France or Dakar. The city's economy, historically based entirely on commerce, faltered throughout the mid-twentieth century and more or less collapsed at independence.

Saint Louis is now, by all accounts, a *dekk bu wow*, or dry city,[1] a term that conveys poverty and fall from political significance. There has been little eco-nomic growth in the forty-five years since independence, and the population has become increasingly impoverished. In spite of this poverty, Saint Louis' population has exploded since independence. Cycles of drought in the Senegal River Valley sparked rural crisis and labor migration to Saint Louis, Dakar, and

Europe. Ironically, Saint Louis became one of the primary destinations of rural migrants seeking relief from harsh conditions just as it experienced its own economic downfall. Male residents of Saint Louis are increasingly migrating elsewhere for work, and self-employment in the informal sector is usually the only option for migrants coming to Saint Louis from the rural areas.

There are several interpretations of Saint Louis' economic stagnation in the postcolonial period. Some scholars mourn the loss of the prestigious French city and decry the ruralization of the former colonial gem. This colonial nostalgia is countered by others who describe the decades after independence as a period of Africanization during which city dwellers managed to survive and maintain a viable urban space despite tremendous economic and political impediments (Bonnardel 1992). Unfortunately, the initial optimism about the potential of OMVS projects in the 1980s and 1990s to bring about Saint Louis' economic recovery has not proved warranted. The city continues to struggle with population growth, flooding, and an inability to maintain the existing infrastructure or expand it to serve a growing population.

Postindependence Decline

The end of Saint Louis' economic and administrative importance at independence coincided with increased rural migration from the Middle Valley of the Senegal River and an unprecedented population boom: the population nearly tripled between 1960 and 1985. This surge stemmed from population growth among the urban population and heavy migration from the rural areas, especially during severe droughts in 1968 and 1973. The combination of rising poverty and population growth led to a process referred to by one geographer as the ruralization of the city, as rural migrants created villages, or *bidonvilles*, at the peripheries of town in places like Pikine and Goxumbaaj (Camera 1968).[2]

One of the most important aspects of Saint Louis' recent history has been the inability of urban planning and development to cope with population growth. Environmental limitations, such as the small size of the island and the swampy Senegal River Delta, have created unique challenges to urban development. This population pressure facilitated the establishment of unplanned or chaotic neighborhoods like Pikine that were created by city residents, not by city planners (Ndiaye 1987). Over time new neighborhoods moved closer and closer to swampy areas of the mainland and to the river's floodplains. By the 1980s the surface area of these "spontaneous" urban neighborhoods exceeded that of the planned urban areas (Bonnardel 1992, 337). The consequences of Saint Louis' population growth include high population densities, illegal occupation of public spaces (such as streets), and very unbalanced development, with 51 percent of the city's infrastructure located on the island, where only 17 percent of the city's residents live (Boye 1984; Spierenberg et al. 1999).

Although the 1984 development plan offered suggestions for decongesting the most populated areas and reorganizing chaotic neighborhoods such as Pikine, little progress has been made over the past two decades. In recent years the region of Saint Louis has been marked by increasing poverty, drought, and rural exodus, all of which have exacerbated the problem of demographic pressure on limited urban space (Spierenberg et al. 1999). In addition to its inability to manage high rates of growth, the municipality is plagued by sanitation problems, especially the removal of wastewater and trash. The absence of a reliable sanitation system and chronic flooding create hygiene hazards for most Saint Louis residents. These problems coupled with the inadequacy of the health care system pose serious challenges for the medical district and for residents themselves. The city built a dyke at the southern end of the city to mitigate the worst of the annual flooding, and there are indications that the plans to privatize land and reorganize Pikine are underway. These signs of progress are encouraging to some city residents, but most remain pessimistic that the city will ever have adequate resources to provide services to its population of 250,000.

In spite of the attempts to develop the Senegal River Valley, tourism is the only growing industry that has had a positive effect on Saint Louis' economy. Throughout the 1990s, as the civil war in the Casamance (Senegal's primary tourist destination) continued, Saint Louis became an alternative destination for European vacationers. A significant number of restaurants, hostels, casinos, art galleries, travel agencies, and nightclubs opened, and the tourist sector continues to expand, with new resort hotels being built along the Atlantic coast. European expatriates own most of these businesses, so it is difficult to assess their economic benefit to the Senegalese. Many of the registered tour guides who work for the city's tourism board have earned B.A.s or M.A.s from the University of Saint Louis, which suggests that the tourism industry offers the only possibility of employment for many of Saint Louis' most educated residents.

There is a severe employment crisis in Saint Louis as elsewhere in Senegal; only a small percentage of Saint Louisiens find work in the formal sector. Commercial fishing remains the most productive economic niche in Saint Louis although it has undergone a period of crisis since the 1980s. Whereas in the 1960s Saint Louis supplied most of the fish consumed in the Peanut Basin, now local fisherman compete with those in Kayar, Dakar, and Mbour. The vast majority of Saint Louis' residents are employed in the informal sector, mainly running microbusinesses or small restaurants or food stands. In the early 1990s Bonnardel estimated that about 10,000 women were involved in microcommerce (Bonnardel 1992, 282), and this is easily observable in Saint Louis today. These women have limited amounts of capital and their daily profits are minimal, sometimes less than the price of the main family meal ($2). Nonetheless, microbusinesses are often the only means of survival for many women, especially those whose husbands have no regular employment.

Pikine: Bidonville par Excellence?

One sign of Saint Louis' transformation since 1960 is the deterioration of the prestigious buildings and residences on the island, many of which have fallen into ruin, while the periphery of the city has experienced rapid, unplanned urban growth resulting in neighborhoods that are typically described as bidonvilles or shantytowns. Dwellings in these new urban areas range from huts with thatch roofs to wooden slat houses or cement houses. In these neighborhoods there are no streets or sidewalks, no building codes, limited access to water and electricity, and there is little to no medical or educational infrastructure. Pikine typifies these new, chaotic neighborhoods; in the 1960s it became the primary destination for overcrowded city dwellers and rural migrants seeking relief from drought. Pikine covers about 40 hectares at the southern periphery of Saint Louis, and many of its dwellings were built in the Senegal River's floodplain.

Pikine's growth rate is estimated to be 9 to 10 percent per year, and population estimates were about 45,000 in 1999, or about 30 percent of the total population of Saint Louis with only a fraction of the city's public infrastructure (Ndiaye 1987; Spierenberg et al. 1999). After nearly thirty years of drought, the rains are returning to predrought levels, creating near annual flooding throughout much of Saint Louis. During the summer of 1999 many Pikine residents were housed in tents along the highway leading into town for more than two months while they waited for the flooding to recede.

One of the most striking aspects of Saint Louis' urban development is that the neighborhoods with the highest population densities have the least infrastructure; Pikine presents a remarkable case of marginalization and bias in urban planning. In spite of being home to 30 percent of the city's residents, Pikine has only two schools and a single dispensary (with one nurse). Pikine consistently ranks last among Saint Louis neighborhoods by the following criteria: fewest residents living in modern houses, fewest houses with running water, fewest houses with toilets connected to a sewer system, and fewest houses with electricity (in spite of the presence of an electric plant in Pikine) (Houma 1993).

While Pikine shares its marginal status with the other neighborhoods in Saint Louis, its designation as a *quartier non-loti*, or unorganized neighborhood, presents particular problems. Basic issues such as access to water, electricity, a sanitation system, and trash removal cannot be addressed, according to city officials, until Pikine is divided into plots and homeowners can demonstrate that they are in legal possession of their property. The rapid and haphazard settlement of Pikine over the past fifty years, exacerbated by the use of verbal land contracts and rental agreements, created the current situation in which it is virtually impossible for most residents to prove they are legally in possession of the property they occupy.

The theoretical solution to Pikine's chaotic development is lotissement, the complete rezoning of the neighborhood. This process would involve tracing new roads and public recreation areas, relocating households currently residing in these areas, and registering all property owners and giving them deeds to their land. Lotissement would also allow for the installation of infrastructure such as lighting, more public water fountains, and a sewage system. Numerous feasibility studies have been conducted in attempts to develop the plans for Pikine's restructuring. One project in the 1970s was discussed for a period of roughly eight years before it was abandoned because of incomplete documentation to implement the rezoning plan.

In the 1990s another lostissement project was sponsored by Fonds Européens pour le Développement (FED) and GTZ, a German development agency. Originally conceived of as a two-year project, the Pikine Project lasted more than five years, and no significant results were achieved. Elaborate plans were drawn up for the new Pikine, complete with mosques, schools, health facilities, roads, and so on. These plans were on display throughout my field research period in the urbanism office on the island, unbeknownst to most Pikine residents. In the late 1990s surveying teams could be seen in Pikine, and residents were more or less familiar with the plans, but most of them remained skeptical. Finally in the summer of 2006 efforts began to move Pikine residents from areas designated for new roads or public spaces, and the first wave of monetary compensations for these relocations had begun.

The current lack of infrastructure in Pikine also affects individual households. At the time of the last household survey, 40 percent of Pikine households had electricity and 50 percent had a water tap (Ly 1997). Households without a water tap obtain water from the public fountains located throughout the neighborhood. Sixty two percent of Pikine houses had a toilet connected to a septic system, and 8 percent had latrines (Ly 1997). Households without toilets or latrines dump their waste in the river; many unoccupied spaces have become public trash dumps for household waste. The most common dumping areas are along the riverbanks and near the flood basin. One popular dumping site is adjacent to the Pikine dispensary. This creates numerous problems with hygiene even during the dry season, and during the flood of 1999 this area was completely inundated and garbage continued to rot in the floodwater.

Because of limited educational opportunities, most Pikine children drop out of elementary school after a few years and seek work in the informal sector. Pikine has the dubious distinction of supplying more maids to the city than any other neighborhood (Ndiaye 1987). The few children in school and the lack of any recreational facilities fosters delinquency, drug use, and prostitution among Pikine youth. Pikine is home to the majority of taxi drivers, public transport drivers, and the young male fare collectors who work in teams with the drivers. The thriving informal sector in Pikine employs many residents and attracts blue-collar workers from other neighborhoods and from rural areas. Most women engage in some kind of small trade or petty commerce, such as selling produce from a small table in front of their homes or even on a small cloth spread out on the ground. Women also sell snack food items such as fried doughnuts or roasted peanuts, but their profits tend to be minuscule.

Pikine residents maintain a sense of defiant pride in their neighborhood in spite of its many problems and their resentment of local authorities. There have been several attempts to organize at the grassroots level to confront the neighborhood problems of flooding and trash. Periodic attempts occur to clean up trash depots, and residents once organized themselves to build a foot bridge across the flood basin. These efforts tend to enjoy moderate success for a time but are not sustainable without infrastructure and support from city government. Attempts to resolve local problems belie the stereotypes of Pikine residents as lazy, uneducated, or incompetent compared with their bourgeois neighbors on the island. In spite of the desire of many Pikinois to develop their neighborhood, political wrangling within Pikine hampers these efforts. The once successful Pikine Development Association eventually fell into obscurity because of political competition among neighborhood notables.

The elusive promise of lotissement served as the justification for city officials' neglect of Pikine throughout the 1990s, particularly in the domain of public health infrastructure. In Saint Louis as throughout Senegal, malaria is a main cause of morbidity and mortality. Chronic problems with flooding and standing water in Pikine during the rainy season, coupled with inadequate housing, make the population extremely vulnerable (Ministère de la Santé et de la Prevention Médicale 2006). Many of Pikine's health problems such as malnutrition are closely linked to poverty, but the lack of universal access to clean water, sanitation, and waste removal also pose great challenges to promoting health in Pikine. Even in the absence of additional medical resources, such as more clinics and more medical staff, improvements in public health would undoubtedly reduce rates of diarrhea, parasites, and infectious diseases. Given the ongoing trend of state withdrawal from social services and the inability of local government to maintain the limited infrastructure already in existence, it seems unlikely that Pikine's problems will be resolved in the near future.

Living in Development's Shadow: Changing Economies in Ganjool

The area south of Saint Louis along the Senegal River Delta is made up of a stretch of villages referred to collectively as Ganjool. Despite the seeming geographical and social distance between the former colonial capital and this region, much of which is without access to electricity, phone service, or running water, there have been economic and political links between these zones since the earliest days of colonial conquest. In recent years with the declining agricultural productivity of Ganjool's soils, more and more Ganjool residents have migrated to Saint Louis to seek other economic opportunities. Most of them are now residents of Pikine, and there is daily traffic between Ganjool and Pikine as members of the Ganjool diaspora attend major social events (weddings, baptisms, and funerals) in their villages of origin and rural dwellers come to town for similar events.

Since its settlement several centuries ago, Ganjool's economy has been based on the cultivation of crops such as manioc, millet, sweet potatoes and potatoes, tomatoes, cucumbers, watermelon and local melons, and groundnuts. Early residents were attracted to the shallow water tables and freshwater wells that allowed for the cultivation of both rain-fed and hand-irrigated crops. There was also plenty of vegetation to maintain herds of cattle, camels, and donkeys. The past thirty or so years of drought that have affected all of northern Senegal have greatly reduced the vegetation needed to sustain these herds, but many households in Ganjool had camels through the 1970s. Communal fishing was more common than hunting, and the local salt mines historically supplied the entire region with salt.

The precolonial Wolof kingdoms have received substantial treatment in the historiography of Senegal, but the history of the Ganjool region remains for the most part unwritten. Caught between the competing authorities of the *damel* of Cajoor and the *brak* of Waalo (both precolonial kingdoms), Ganjool appears briefly as an aside in the histories of these kingdoms by Barry (1972), Diouf (1990), and Witherell (1964).[3] Of particular interest to both the damel and the brak of Waalo were Ganjool's salt mines, which reportedly produced 20,000 French francs of revenue annually in the mid-nineteenth century (Diagne 1919).[4] Ganjool was one of the first regions of Cajoor to become part of the French "enclave" around the base of operations in Saint Louis. In the period before the railroad was built through the heart of peanut production in Cajoor, Ganjool was the main *entrepôt* where peanuts were brought from the interior and sold to the French (Witherell 1964). Besides the conflicts over salt mines, the pillaging of French shipwrecks, and the service of Ganjool's camel riders on French missions, little of the story of Ganjool's early settlement, expansion, and ongoing relationship with the French colony in Saint Louis has been documented.

Daru-Mumbaay

Daru-Mumbaay is located along the coast of the Senegal River, a few kilometers south of one of the three original Ganjool villages called Muid. Its current population is roughly 1,200 full and part-time residents who make up around 110 households. There are no written records of the village's founding, but the village chief and one of his peers, both in their late eighties, told me similar stories about how the village was created. As the village of Muid continued to expand at the turn of the twentieth century, population pressure spurred many people to move farther inland and south along the coast of the Senegal River to found satellite villages. The villages of Daru and Mumbaay each started as part of this expansion from Muid, and they eventually merged to become Daru-Mumbaay.

Today the village is organized into several small neighborhoods that are referred to by derivations of names of the first families to settle there. These include Ngeyeen (from the last name Gey), Jooben (from Joob), and Niangeen (from Niang). At the heart of the village are small boutiques on both sides of the road, the village school, the health hut, and the market. In recent years a credit agency opened up where villagers with collateral (typically men who own land) can secure small business loans. This central area serves as a sort of village square, and here one finds the *grand place* where young and old men spend their leisure time under the shade of trees and open-air shelters. The *grand place* is most animated from about 11 a.m. until the main meal at 2 P.M. Men also gather in the late afternoon and do their evening prayers there (5 P.M. and 7 P.M.). Women have no such designated leisure spot and have much less leisure time, but they usually chat and exchange information in the market and at the machine, the petrol-operated mill where women grind millet into flour.

Most of the village neighborhoods have their own small mosques (*jakaa*) where residents perform their daily prayers. The large mosque (*jumaa*) is used only on Fridays and is equipped with a battery-powered public address system that broadcasts the call to prayer. Typically only men and older women attend the Friday prayer. This PA system is also used to announce deaths in Daru-Mumbaay and in neighboring villages. The PA system is always an unwelcome sound on any day but Friday, and it was a constant reminder of misfortune during the rainy season of 1999 when a number of people died in the course of a few weeks.

South of the jumaa are the neighborhoods of Jooben and Ngeyeen. The main footpath from the road into these neighborhoods is designated "Islam corner" by a small wooden side next to the small mosque just off the road. The combined area of Jooben and Ngeyeen has about twenty-two households and a population of approximately two hundred people. I resided in Ngeyeen through-out my stay in the village, and I knew the families in Jooben and Ngeyeen the most intimately because of our close proximity. Just south of Ngeyeen are the houses of some Mauritanian families (called *naar* by the Wolof). Mumbaay is predominantly Wolof, but there are small clusters of Haalpulaar families all along the main north-south axis that cuts through Ganjool.

Changing Economies: From Farming to Fishing

From the late nineteenth century through the 1970s, many residents of Ganjool kept herds of camels, cattle, sheep, and goats. Traditionally Ganjool was an area where pastoralists from Waalo and Cajoor would bring their herds for grazing during the dry season, but its extensive forest areas and vegetation have been irreparably damaged by drought and accompanying desertification of the past forty years. When collecting information about men's labor histories, I found that one of the major occupations of men only a generation ago, *jëgg* (transporting goods by camel), had disappeared due to the changes in transportation and the near impossibility of maintaining herds of animals on sparse vegetation.

Fishing and farming remain the principal occupations of most men in Daru-Mumbaay. A few men with sufficient start-up capital have managed to open small shops or to work as *bana-bana*, traveling merchants who buy goods in one part of the country and sell them in another. There are several men who own horse carts and provide transportation to neighboring villages and also transport produce to area markets. Many boys combine attending school with working in their parents' fields in the off-season, or before their morning classes during the main farming season. Some men combine farming with bricklaying or river fishing. The advantage of nonfarming occupations is the possibility of earning a small income every day, as opposed to living on credit for much of the year and then trying to pay off debts at harvest time. The few men who fish in the river are able to use the day's catch to meet their expenses, and so they avoid accumulating the large debts that plague the farmers who "go to work in the fields every day and come home without a dime in their pockets." They are also able to take days off or travel when necessary, whereas missing even a day or two of watering could threaten to ruin an onion crop.

Although onion farming has been the dominant economic strategy in Daru-Mumbaay for the past several decades, the quality of soils and the profits from red onions have been steadily declining. Most residents do not have a clear understanding of how the anti-salt dam at Diama operates, but they recognize that the farming crisis began after the dam opened in 1988. The negative effects of the dam on the Senegal River Delta, mainly due to salinization of soils and the water table, were anticipated by scholars and some development agents (Adams 2000). Local farmers describe the changes of the past decade in terms of declining yields, wells that have gone salty, and an inescapable cycle of debt in which the year's harvest is not enough to cover the year's expenses. One farmer explains the recent changes:

> Things have changed. What has changed is that the fields used to be good. Whatever you planted, it would grow. Now we plant our seedlings and nothing happens; nothing takes in the soil. Where you used to get twenty onions now you get only ten. The soil doesn't have any strength left. . . . There are lots of fields that had good wells and now the water is no good. And you know all of those crops need freshwater, like beans,

they need a good place to grow. I remember one year Mor Sen's field, the one next to mine, there was one year when he grew beans and it was unbelievable. But today if you went to that field you couldn't get anything to grow. You can go gather salt there. The water is no good. . . . And every year it gets worse.

The environmental damage that Ganjool has experienced over the past decade has made it exceedingly difficult for farmers to earn a profit from onions. As onions were a lucrative crop in the past, many of the farmers working the new irrigated perimeters in the Middle Senegal Valley are now growing them. This new competition from the valley combined with environmental damage has been disastrous for Ganjool's farmers.

For the past twenty years, even in a year with a seemingly good harvest, the debts that a farmer accumulates during the growing season are nearly impossible to repay. This cycle of debt coupled with the fall in the profitability of onions has been a shock to Ganjool's economy and a source of distress, particularly for male heads of households. To avoid this cycle of poverty and debt, many young men have abandoned farming altogether to seek their fortune through travel or fishing in the Gambia. It would be difficult to overstate this rapid transition from farming to fishing as an economic strategy. Almost any boy under the age of ten will say that when he grows up he wants to go to the Gambia to fish. These boys and young men have watched their parents farming year after year without attaining financial security. In contrast, they see fishermen (mool) return from their ten-month stint in the Gambia in wooden fishing boats loaded with merchandise. Young boys who apprentice themselves to experienced fishermen might become captains after a few fishing seasons, and they gradually earn enough money to purchase a boat. Once they own a boat men can get married, build a house, or invest their profits by buying additional boats. While men who farm typically experience difficulty saving the necessary brideprice to get married, their mool counterparts are often able to afford marriage in their early to mid-twenties.

Men's labor histories reveal that the transition to fishing has occurred within the past generation, and only younger men have been able to pursue this new strategy. Nearly all of the migrant fisherman are younger than thirty five. Once men reach the age of thirty they are most likely married and have children, which requires a daily financial contribution for the household's meals (referred to colloquially as the DQ, dépenses quotidiennes). It becomes increasingly difficult to make the transition to fishing as they cannot leave their wives and children without support for ten months. Several men in their thirties expressed regret that it was "too late" for them to go to work as mool, and they had resigned themselves to a lifetime of hard work and debt as farmers. Mustafa Joob, himself a fisherman who does not migrate but instead fishes in the river and has all but abandoned farming, explains: "The older you get the less farming you do, because it demands a lot of strength. Lots of people don't have a choice; they don't have any other kind of work to do. But all of the people who are here farming, it's not their first choice. They don't have anything else, so they farm no matter how hard it is. All the ones who are still farming, it's because they do not have a choice." The worst of a limited number of options, farming has come to be viewed as a last resort.

The relatively new trend of migration to the Gambia has had dramatic effects on Daru-Mumbaay, the most noticeable of which is the absence of over half of the male population between the ages of ten and thirty-five. In many households all of the sons have migrated, and some women and children spend nine or ten months of the year waiting for the return of their husbands and fathers. Household economies have changed as fathers have lost the labor of many of their sons. Traditionally, young men would work for their fathers until they were old enough to marry; the fathers would give them a portion of their harvest earnings, keeping the rest to help manage household expenses. Now boys as young as ten or twelve work the boats of their older siblings or cousins and keep most of the profits they are paid at the end of the fishing season for themselves. This loss of their sons' labor explains some of the trips that older men in the village make to the Gambia to visit the mool. Many are given gifts of cash before they return home, and others spend the entire fishing season in the Gambia working as fishmongers.

Some women and children accompany the migrants to the Gambia, but the transition to fishing has largely been a male phenomenon. Women in Mumbaay have very limited options for earning money. Most girls begin helping their mothers by the age of six or seven, the age at which they become responsible for a number of domestic chores such as washing dishes, supervising younger siblings, and doing the daily marketing. By the time they are teenagers or young adults, girls can make substantial contributions to the household economy with their agricultural labor. They will usually be given a small amount of their total earnings, and their parents will use the rest to buy them clothes and to help with other household expenses.

After marriage, women's first responsibility is to take care of domestic chores such as meal preparation, cleaning, and child care. Most women farm small plots during onion season, and they might also have kitchen gardens where they grow green onions and other condiments. They rely on their husbands or fathers for access to land, and must reimburse them (or another creditor) for seed, fertilizers, and pesticides. Once they have paid these debts, they maintain control over their earnings. There is no joint account for the household; husbands and wives take charge of their own earnings. Husbands are responsible for providing their dependents with food, clothing, and shelter, so women use their earnings to supplement the money their husbands give them for household expenses.

A handful of women in Daru Mumbaay have achieved moderate success as traders or bana-bana. Most are over the age of fifty and they have relinquished their domestic responsibilities to adult daughters, younger co-wives, or their daughters-in-law. These women acquired enough capital to begin traveling to local markets with produce from Ganjool to sell, or they travel to Mauritania and other locations where they can obtain sugar, soap, and other products at wholesale prices. A more common strategy for women, and usually a less successful one, is to sell small items such as snack foods in the village market or in their immediate neighborhood. A few of my neighbors tried to start a business selling fried bean cakes, but their production schedule was erratic and their profit margin was very small. Another neighbor bought several kilos of raw peanuts, which she then roasted and gave to her ten-year-old daughter to sell (giving her strict instructions not to sell on credit). She attempted to sell peanuts for a few weeks and then decided the minuscule profits were not worth the addition to her already heavy workload. Most women who start these kinds of microbusinesses have only a few dollars of start-up capital and might earn the equivalent of twenty-five or fifty cents a day. Most of their potential customers are as strapped for cash as they are, which makes it even more difficult to maintain a successful business.

Although there are few occupational niches in Mumbaay, there are important differences in social status and economic security among households. One of the most important status considerations is length of residency in the village. In spite of the declining profits from red onions, many men migrate from poorer regions of Senegal to sell their labor to landowners who provide them with room and board and a share in the harvest profits. Many of the poorer households were established when these wage laborers, referred to as *suurga* (strangers) decided to stay in the village permanently. These individuals are less embedded in the complex village genealogies, and their family histories are less well known than those of the founding families.[5] Many remain poor and somewhat marginalized even after several generations.

When I conducted interviews asking about economic stratification in the village, people responded with four main categories pertaining to food security. In the top category are well-off or comfortable families. They were described as easily meeting their household's daily food needs, that is, "they don't struggle with the DQ." Forty-six households are in this category (approximately 38 percent). Within this top tier is a further distinction between those who are truly wealthy (sixteen families) versus those who are comfortable but not wealthy (twenty-five families).[6]

In the second tier are households that are just barely able to meet their daily food needs. These thirty households (25 percent of the village) were considered to be struggling to make ends meet. The third category consisted of twenty junior males who are still members of their fathers' households. The majority of these men are mool in the Gambia or are working as traders, and thus are wellplaced for financial success. However, they are still seen as part of their fathers' households, and thus their financial situation can't yet be assessed. Finally, in the bottom category are twenty-six households (21 percent) described as being unable to meet their household food needs; they are occasionally or even frequently forced to skip meals. The households in each category are distributed relatively evenly among the main village neighborhoods.

Although the sample size is quite small, when wealth-ranking data are compared with men's occupations several patterns emerge. Of the sixteen wealthiest households in the village, nine heads of household are either traders or boutique owners. Although a few of these merchants combine business with farming, there are no men in this category who have achieved financial success by farming alone. In the other subgroup of this top category there are ten farmers who are comfortable but not wealthy. This pattern suggests that in the best cases farming allows one to attain household food security, but not surplus wealth. Farmers are in the majority among households that are struggling and those that are missing meals, but there is no clear indication of why some farmers achieve food security and others do not. Many different variables such as the field size and quality, and the number of adults and children in a given household, might account for some of this variation.

The Rhythm of Daily Life: Work and Play

In spite of the notable rise in male migration, life in Mumbaay still revolves around the red onion (sonsaa) season, which starts in December when men and women plant seedbeds. Seedlings will be watered for approximately two months and then transplanted into the fields in February. Once transplanted, the seedlings must be watered every day. Watering is a grueling activity that involves throwing a bucket attached to a long rope into a well that is four to ten meters deep and pulling the bucket out of the well in a rapid hand-over-hand motion. When two buckets have been filled, the farmer walks between the rows of onion plants emptying a bucket with each hand. Speed and strength to lift the buckets or rubber bags from the well are the most important factors in successful onion farming.

Although the sonsaa plants thrive in heat and sandy soil, missing even a day of watering could jeopardize them, thus the four-month period of watering is a demanding trial for men and women. One farmer describes a typical day in the onion fields: "When I am in the middle of sonsaa season, most of the time I get up at 5 A.M. I will go to the fields at 5 A.M. and work until noon or 1 P.M. I come back to the house and lie down and rest. After I eat lunch and drink tea, I will go back to the fields. I will weed or I will take the pump and use insecticide. I will work until 6 or 7 P.M. and then come home and rest. Once I have eaten dinner, there is no going out again or walking around, I go straight to bed. When it is 5 A.M. I go to work again. That's how it is until the onions are ready to be harvested." The average workday for most men during the sonsaa season is approximately eleven hours of grueling physical labor.

Although women are much less ambitious in the amount of seedlings they will transplant and water, they must combine an already heavy domestic workload with the unrelenting watering schedule. Women make a convincing argument that although they plant fewer seedlings than men, they work as hard or harder than the men do: "Women in Ganjool, during sonsaa they are more tired than men. The men go to the fields in the morning, and when they come back they can lie down and rest until the afternoon. They don't have anything else they have to do in the house. But women, we have to combine farming with all of the housework." The combination of child care, domestic labor, and working in the fields results in workdays that are easily twelve or fourteen hours for many women. My neighbor Jeynaba, who had several children under the age of six, described the basic routine for most women:

> When you get up, after you have prayed, you sweep. Then you wash your baby's clothes. You know if you have a small child, every day you have to wash their diapers. It isn't the same as when you have older children. If you have work to do in the fields you go. You wear your baby on your back and you water your fields. You know that kind of work is hard. If you don't have anyone to take care of your child, you wear him on your back. Then I go to the market, get my ingredients, and light the fire for lunch. Then I cook lunch and we eat lunch and I wash out my bowls. I go take a bath and then I give my children a bath and dress them. If it is this time of year you don't cook dinner because you are tired. When you are in the middle of sonsaa season, the real work, your butt doesn't ever touch the ground until it is time to go to bed. You get up in the morning and you work until night and your butt never touches the ground.

Most extended families assist each other during the intense labor bottlenecks of transplanting the seedlings and again during the harvest when the onion plants must be cut, sorted, and bagged for transport to market. Women described these two phases of the agricultural cycle as especially difficult because every day they are trying to work in their own fields and participate in the collective work efforts in neighboring fields. Beyond being intensive in its own right, the labor demands on women during sonsaa season also prevented them from having time to respond to bouts of family illness. All but the most urgent complaints are brushed aside as women simply have no time or energy to visit medical practitioners.

In spite of their tenacity and their claim that they work as hard or harder than men, women also feel that farming is truly men's work.

We women of Ganjool, we don't have a choice. If we had a choice we wouldn't be farming. We would be doing some other kinds of women's work. Because farming is men's work. When you are throwing the bags into the well, and putting your hands around that narrow rope, the bucket weighs 5 kilos. You put a rope on it and a stick and you are pulling it up out of the well and watering, and if you have a small child you are wearing that child on your back, you are carrying ten kilos, five kilo buckets in each hand filled with water, and then you go and pour it out and come back and get more. And if you are a woman you will do it two hundred times, women do it two hundred times in a day. If it was a man, they do it four hundred times or five hundred times.

The difficult labor of pulling the buckets up hand over hand out of relatively deep wells leaves men and women exhausted long before the end of the sonsaa season. Everyone suffers from various ailments related to fatigue and overwork. As Awa Joob says, "Watering sonsaa is really awful. It is hard for women. Once you are doing it you don't even look like a person anymore." At the end of the long growing season when everyone is in the village square weighing and selling their onions, they commiserate about their aching bodies and maladies. "You go to the market and no one is well. They say, 'I am rotten, I have melted.'" Even in a good year, most people reason that onion farming is not worth the strenuous labor necessary to produce the crop, but with few alternatives it is seen as the only option.

After four months of steady watering, sonsaa onions are harvested in midsummer. Most farmers try to wait until they will get the best price at the market, and once the onions are full size they can be left in the ground for several weeks. If they are not harvested before the first rains fall, however, they risk getting soggy and spoiling. When the onion harvest has been successful, the residents of Mumbaay can look forward to three or four months of leisure time and weddings. The village masons will be busy building for those who have earned enough money to add rooms to their compounds. Only a few crops are grown during the rainy season, and they do not require as intensive a schedule of watering and weeding. From June through September, most men's workdays will be shortened to five or six hours. This is the season when men come back from the fields by 10:30 or 11 a.m. and populate the *grand place* until lunchtime.

Women's workloads also decrease, although they are still occupied much of the time with their domestic labor. During the rainy season from June or July to September, the river changes from "bitter" to "sweet" and children spend much of the day swimming and playing on the river banks. Once the water is no longer salty, most men and women will take their afternoon bath in the river. This period of downtime also permits other kinds of activities that people find too exhausting during sonsaa season. These special events range from midnight wrestling matches accompanied by *sabar* drums to performances by the village theater troupe.

One of the regular social activities that occurs even during the sonsaa season is a gathering that is referred to as a *tuur*. Tuur take place every Saturday, with women's tuur at around 5 P.M. and men's tuur at about 8 P.M. The membership of any given tuur is similar to an age-grade association; it is made up of approximately ten to fifteen men or women in the same peer group. A different member hosts the tuur each week and is required to provide tea, biscuits or peanuts, and sometimes a version of Kool-Aid for the rest of the members. Small dues are paid weekly to help the host or hostess pay for the tuur, and fines can also be given if a person arrives late. These tuur are scaled-back versions of the same kind of phenomenon that takes place in Saint Louis and Dakar. At the urban tuur the dues can be quite high ($10 and up as opposed to a few cents), and most hostesses will rent stereo equipment and sometimes pay a disc jockey. At some tuur the focus is on music and dancing, and prizes will often be awarded to the most skilled and provocative dancers. Village tuur infrequently have music, but are always animated by a rousing exchange of local gossip and other news. These weekly social gatherings proved to be a useful place to collect data on local happenings and on women's views about health challenges and medical strategies.

Urban and Rural Dilemmas Compared

Although the daily experiences of residents of Ganjool and Pikine are quite different, they face similar challenges coping with the economic challenges of the past twenty years. Gender, age, generation, and geographic location have mediated these economic changes, creating new possibilities for some but not others. The city of Saint Louis has been striving unsuccessfully to develop new economic sectors, and Pikine represents the empty promise of urban life for the thousands of migrants who have arrived in Senegal's city and towns hoping to escape rural poverty. Even a brief visit to Pikine offers a view of the dismal living conditions of the many residents who live in cramped housing, wait in line for hours to obtain water for household needs, and move quietly under the cover of darkness to dispose of household waste near the river. The nearly annual flooding of the Senegal River, whose floodplains reach the center of Pikine, ironically turns individuals fleeing cycles of rural drought into water refugees whose houses are submerged under standing water for weeks at a time. Most of the day and well into the evening one finds men of all ages loitering around small boutiques, lounging on benches under shade trees, listening to the radio, and heatedly discussing local and national politics. Their presence is a reminder of the exceedingly high unemployment rates and the saturated informal labor market. The gendered division of labor provides women with more opportunities to work in the informal market as they can turn their domestic skills of cooking, cleaning, washing laundry, and marketing into income-generating activities on a full- or part-time basis. The increase in tourism has also expanded the market for sex work and other transactional exchanges with male tourists.

Ganjool's economic downturn is equally problematic as the recent environmental degradation has devastated local agricultural production and plunged many farmers into seemingly irreversible debt. The decreasing returns on onion farming have increased household economic insecurity with numerous effects on generational and gendered relations. The absence of young men aged fifteen to thirty-five has affected not only the social climate in the village, but marriage and residence patterns and household relations of production. Senior men can no longer count on the earning power of their male dependents as the latter are increasingly taking charge of their own labor by leaving the village. While a few senior women become successful traders, there are very few options for young women besides farming and marriage. Young people in the city and the village dream of escaping the limitations of their present circumstances. While young men in Ganjool launch their fishing boats every season to head to the rich fishing zones of the Cap Vert region, these same boats made international headlines when hundreds of young men from Saint Louis and other towns lost their lives as they attempted to survive for weeks at sea on their way to Spain via the Canary Islands. When I visited the village in 2008, I learned that two of the young men in my household had successfully made the voyage to Spain, and that one had traveled as far as Italy where he is now living with a cousin.

Rural and urban variations on economic distress form the backdrop against which individuals and families attempt to respond to illness and promote health. Vulnerability to disease stems from food insecurity, flooding, and irregular access to clean water, which are shared problems across the rural-urban divide. For shantytown dwellers in Pikine, high population densities, lack of a sewage system, and the ubiquitous dumping of waste in public spaces bring additional threats to public health. The difficult labor of onion farming paired with insufficient caloric intake leaves many Ganjool farmers anemic and subject to extreme fatigue and exhaustion. These are the sorts of inequalities that become written on the body in the form of affliction and suffering (Farmer 2005).

Both Ganjool and Pikine lack sufficient infrastructure, particularly medical infrastructure. Pikine's most obvious problem is the lack of medical personnel—there is just one nurse for a population of 50,000. Pikine residents complained most consistently about the poor quality of care and inaccessible location of their health post. The head nurse of the health post had an extremely poor reputation, and residents often assumed if they tried to visit the health post they would find it closed, the nurse would be missing, or there would be no vaccinations and no drugs. During my research, each of these occurrences was indeed a distinct possibility on any given day, which meant that many Pikine residents frequented health posts in other neighborhoods or went directly to the hospital.

Although Daru-Mumbaay has only a health hut and two community health workers, most villagers were more concerned about the limited possibilities for rapid transportation to the Saint Louis hospital in case of a medical emergency. The past decade has seen steady deterioration of the paved road from Tassinère to Saint Louis, and the entire road was underwater for many weeks during the floods of 1999. The road from Daru-Mumbaay to Tassinère, the location of Ganjool's health post, is unpaved and often impassable during the rainy season. Families in Daru-Mumbaay agreed that it would be a tremendous advantage to have their own nurse and health post in the village, but the difficulty of evacuating gravely ill patients was a more pressing problem.

Saint Louis, Pikine, and Ganjool have each been affected by shifts in the regional political economy, and the state's vision of development (or lack thereof) for the Senegal River Valley and the river delta. The commercial decline of Saint Louis at independence coupled with rural flight created the context for the rise of unplanned neighborhoods like Pikine. The failed development projects of the OMVS have threatened Ganjool's agricultural economy and sparked waves of labor migration. These outcomes stem largely from social, political, and economic trends that are internal to Senegal. In the following chapter we will examine the encounter between globally driven economic and health policies and Senegal's health system, and how this encounter has shaped the therapeutic landscape in the Saint Louis region.

4

Global Health Reform in Saint Louis

When I moved to Saint Louis in the fall of 1998, I found that most technical personnel working in neighborhood health posts, and the majority of people seeking health care at government health clinics, had little idea what decentralization and the "new health codes" were all about. New financing systems were in place, as were new modes of management at local clinics, yet only the senior administrators in the medical district seemed to have a sense of how the reformed health system was supposed to function. The buzzwords of the reforms included "community management," "participation," and "state-citizen partnerships for health." A colleague in Dakar whom I interviewed in the first weeks of my fieldwork offered the following assessment:

> There is a whole new equation that people are learning to live with out there. You are coming at a time when it is very much in a state of transformation and fluctuation, where people are just learning how to deal with it. In some cases they are discovering that people who have been given certain responsibilities need additional training in order to be able to do it. They are finding that medical people aren't really prepared to work with community groups and they need training to do that, and they need to learn how to do that without getting on their high horse and saying "I'm the doctor, don't tell me what to do!"

He argued that in spite of the profound changes brought about by decades of structural adjustment and the currency devaluation of 1994, decentralization had a larger impact on the health sector than any other reform of the previous decade.

This assessment of the importance of decentralization vis-à-vis economic reforms surprised me. From the early 1990s to the present, much scholarship in critical medical anthropology has been devoted to lambasting neoliberal economic reforms and the efficiency-driven health reforms associated with them. While neoliberalism risks becoming an empty signifier intended to explain all of the devastating economic and social conditions of the developing world, there is much evidence that these policies have exacerbated poverty and weakened fragile health systems. By the late 1990s Senegal had been undergoing structural adjustment programs (SAPs) for nearly two decades and public spending in the social sector had been significantly reduced. While growth in GDP was reaching close to 5 percent in some years, the absolute number of people living in poverty had increased, as had the disparity between rich and poor (Duruflé 1994).

In Senegal as in dozens of countries throughout the developing world, these economic policies set the stage for the reorganization of state health systems, often through the implementation of user fees for patients and other elements of privatization (Foley 2001; Schoepf et al. 2000; Turshen 1999). These reforms have been part of global trends in which the basic right to health, as articulated at the Alma Ata conference in 1978, has been superseded by market-based models of health care in which consumers have the right to purchase health services (Janes 2004; Hong 2004; Shaw and Griffin 1995; World Bank 1993). This neoliberal approach to primary health care has been the target of widespread criticism on the part of social scientists concerned with shifting health care costs from nation-states to vulnerable populations (Baer 1996 and 1997; Baer et al. 2004; Farmer 2004 and 2005; Janes and Chuluundorj 2004; Kim et al. 2000; Nguyen and Peschard 2003; Turshen 1999).

While the decline in social spending starved the health system of much-needed resources, it did not fundamentally alter the structure of the health system—this would happen only with decentralization. Implemented together in the 1990s, the Bamako Initiative (Africa's solution for primary health care under SAPs) and decentralization significantly altered the organization of the health sector and the responsibilities of health administrators and medical personnel. Citizens, too, found themselves with new responsibilities, as they were charged with contributing to the management of neighborhood health structures. After situating Senegal's reforms within a broader context of changing trends in global health, and offering an overview of Senegal's burden of disease, this chapter highlights the experiences and dilemmas of medical district personnel and district patients who were "learning to live with it."

From Health for All to User Fees: Shifts in Global Health Policy

Like many developing countries, Senegal implemented a primary health care strategy with the goal of "Health for All by the Year 2000" after the Alma Ata Conference in 1978. This strategy emphasizes equitable access to health care and community participation and is characterized by low-cost, preventative medicine and treatment at dispensaries and rural health centers with a referral system to treatment in secondary and higher levels of care. The basic tenets of primary health care include access, participation, sustainability, and prevention. Primary health care recognizes the numerous social and economic determinants of health, and treats health care as a basic right that governments must provide to their citizens.

The global commitment to primary health care proved to be short-lived. By the late 1980s the World Bank began articulating a new agenda for the health sectors of developing countries. Financing Health Services in Developing Countries (World Bank 1987) attacked universal coverage and argued that care should be offered at a cost to patients, since many citizens in developing countries were able and willing to pay for health care. The Bank's "World Development Report: Investing in Health" (1993) offered a model for restructuring health systems. Although the report underlines the connections between poverty and health, the Bank suggested that economic growth, streamlining government spending on the health sector, and privatization would strengthen health sectors and improve the health of the poor. The report emphasized technical efficiency and a reduced role for government, and equitable access to care was not an explicit concern (Blas and Hearst 2002). International health priorities moved away from primary health care strategies and their implicit assertion that universal free health care is a basic human right.

By the early 1980s African governments were hit with the debt crisis that was affecting the rest of the developing world. Public spending on health declined rapidly and governments were urged to downsize and privatize their health sectors (Turshen 1999; Schoepf et al. 2000). Although most governments maintained primary health care rhetoric in health sector planning, universal free health care became more and more elusive as social sector spending plummeted in the 1980s. Governments essentially shifted the financing of health care to citizens by implementing user fees and other attempts to recover costs in the health sector. SAPs enabled Third World governments to maintain payment schedules on their loans, but in case after case these programs proved catastrophic for the health of the poor, and they worsened the lives of millions of men, women, and children (Cornia 1987; Kim et al. 2000; Sparr 1994; Thomas-Emeagwali 1995).

As part of a continent-wide effort to retain a minimum of health services in the wake of reduced state spending on social sectors, Senegal implemented the Bamako Initiative in the 1990s. This new financing plan, created at the World Health Organization (WHO) and United Nation's Children's Fund (UNICEF)-sponsored Bamako meeting in 1987, was designed to increase the availability of essential medicines and to improve drug procurement systems through resale of pharmaceuticals at health centers (Kanji 1989). The chief component of the Bamako Initiative was a community-financing scheme. Clinics would be stocked with mainly generic medicines that would be sold to patients at low cost. The profits from these medicines and the sale of consultation tickets would cover a significant portion of each clinic's operating costs, thus relieving the state from the burden of fully subsidizing health care. This initiative would also ensure a constant supply of drugs for the most common diseases. The goal of these reforms was to improve the quality of health care while keeping it relatively low-cost, and to ensure a constant supply of medicines in health facilities (UNICEF-WHO 1991).

Senegal's implementation of the Bamako Initiative coincided with more widespread attempts to execute decentralization reforms approved by the national legislature in 1996. Decentralization of the health sector meant that locally elected officials at municipal and regional levels had a new charge to include health spending in their annual budgets. At all levels of the health system medical personnel became the financial managers of revenues generated by user fees and drug sales. Medical personnel, in consultation with the health committees, were charged with establishing priorities for investing these health revenues to meet neighborhood and village health needs.

One UNICEF official described this combined emphasis on fee-for-services and a community role in financial management as an attempt to "democratize the business of primary health care." In light of the undemocratic nature of many health committees, one could argue these reforms are more about business than democratic input from community members. Throughout the implementation phase of the Bamako Initiative, the Senegalese Ministry of Health often referred to this financing approach as "the new partnership between the state and citizens for health quality and equity." This concept of state-citizen partnerships has proven remarkably attractive in health development circles in Senegal. Appeals for "responsibilization", or empowering citizens to take responsibility for their health, both as individuals and as effective participants in civil society organizations, were ubiquitous in Senegal during the implementation of the Bamako Initiative, and they remain part of official state and NGO discourse on overcoming Senegal's health challenges.

These attempts to reorganize Senegal's health system are characteristic of the kinds of policies being carried out throughout the developing world and in countries undergoing post socialist transitions. Health reform, which was initiated in most sub-Saharan African countries in response to the external shocks of the debt crisis and austerity programs, has now become a "global experiment" (Roberts et al. 2004). Many political and economic forces are driving health reform globally, including rising costs, the rising expectations of citizens, and the shrinking capacity of governments to finance health care (Roberts et al. 2004). A burgeoning literature on health reform has developed that ranges from critiques of processes and results thus far (Castro and Singer 2004; Kim et al. 2000), to calls for rethinking equity and the ethical underpinnings of reform

(Blas and Hearst 2002; Evans et al. 2001; Gwatkin 2001; Roberts and Reich 2002), and guidelines for "getting health reform right" (Roberts et al. 2004). Recent scholarship emphasizes the shortcomings of health system models based on advanced capitalist economies in the North, and the numerous shortcomings observed when these systems are transplanted into radically different social, political, and economic contexts (Bloom and Standing 2008).

Health-sector reform describes "a significant, purposeful effort to improve the performance of the health care system" (Roberts et al. 2004, 9). Medical anthropologists and global health scholars have developed frameworks for conceptualizing the processes that lead to good (and bad) health reform, and they have identified a range of useful criteria for evaluating the outcomes of health reform (Castro and Singer 2004; Janes et al. 2006; Roberts et al. 2004). Voices from within the World Bank (Gwatkin 2001) and outside it have argued for equity-driven reforms to replace the efficiency-based reforms that were synonymous with neoliberal economic lending policies of the 1980s and 1990s (Evans et al. 2001; Roberts and Reich 2002; Roberts et al. 2004). Equity in health means that health care resources are allocated according to need, and health services are received according to need (Braveman 1998 in Blas and Hearst 2002). As Janes et al. (2006) argue, equitable access to health care reduces disparities in health outcomes, thereby countering inequities that threaten population health and leave the poor vulnerable to greater impoverishment due to serious illness.

Critical reflections on health policy reveal the moral underpinnings of health reform and question the adequacy of various ethical frameworks for achieving equity. Roberts and Reich (2002) draw attention to three philosophical frameworks that can be employed to analyze ethical dilemmas in public health and health sector reform. Utilitarian strategies focus on outcomes and tend to support policies that will bring the greatest good for the greatest number, regardless of fairness or equity (Roberts and Reich 2002). Liberalism focuses on "rights and opportunities" and therefore emphasizes the "choices" that individuals have as opposed to the consequences of their decisions. Communitarian ethical positions examine policies by questioning whether they align with accepted notions of a good and just society.

In their comprehensive guide to "getting health reform right," Roberts and colleagues argue for an egalitarian liberal position, meaning that they emphasize rights and opportunities, but acknowledge that the right to choose "is meaningless without adequate resources" (Roberts et al. 2004, 49). In the egalitarian liberal framework, everyone has the right to a minimum level of services and resources, which tends to lead to a redistributive approach. This positive right to a minimal level of health could be measured by access to a certain level of care or a minimal health status. The egalitarian liberal position dovetails with some of the more activist stances among critical medical anthropologists, such as that of Paul Farmer. He describes his ethical commitment to putting the last first as a "preferential option for the poor" inspired by the social justice tradition of liberation theology (2005). A similar commitment to a universal, egalitarian liberal standard for access to medical care is evident in the global treatment campaign for AIDS drugs (Smith and Siplon 2006). These ethical positions counter the familiar global double standard of medical care, that is, the notion that because of limited resources in the global South it is unrealistic to expect that its residents should have access to the same standard of medical care as those in the global North.

Most health reform has been grounded in utilitarian frameworks that stress cost-effectiveness and ultimate utility, or deploying health resources to achieve the greatest good for the greatest number of people (i.e., financing a primary health care [PHC] approach). World Bank policies and plans for health sector reform and adjustment in the 1980s met with acute critiques that they were overly utilitarian and efficiency oriented, paying no attention to the social and economic costs of adjustment being borne by the most vulnerable populations in adjusting countries (Gwatkin 2001; UNICEF 1987). There is an emerging consensus among global health scholars that health reforms, when informed by a utilitarian logic to distribute health resources in the most cost-effective manner, still result in health systems plagued by avoidable health inequities. Critics point to numerous failures in health reform to date, including the lack of attention to redistributive justice, in spite of the widespread rhetorical commitment to equity and fairness in health systems (Peter and Evans 2001; Castro and Singer 2004). Even a primary health care approach can exacerbate inequalities; data from several countries indicates that the wealthy may benefit more from PHC than the poor (Gwatkin 2001).

After considering Senegal's epidemiological trends over the past twenty years, the remainder of the chapter considers Senegal's health reform experience. My analysis echoes the assertion of other scholars that health sector reforms need to be judged not by their intentions but by the changes they actually produce (Roberts et al. 2004). In the Senegalese case, reforms based in utilitarian and liberal frameworks can actually exacerbate existing social inequalities and reinforce underlying health inequities.

A Look at the Numbers: Senegal's Epidemiological Profile

I had great difficulty obtaining baseline health data, or any data at all, on the Saint Louis region or medical district for reasons I could not have predicted. Despite obtaining research clearance letters from the Minister of Health, I encountered two main problems collecting health statistics: outright resistance to data sharing, and the paucity of data that existed at the clinic or district level. Armed with my research clearance letters, I easily set appointments with both the *medecin-chef* of the region and the medecin-chef of the Saint Louis medical district soon after my arrival in Saint Louis. I was invited to attend the monthly staff meetings of the district medical personnel, and I was able to introduce myself to the head nurses of all the health posts. After my first meeting I approached the district administrator charged with overseeing primary care. I explained that I wanted to interview him about recent changes in the district's operations and his observations of the implementation of health sector reform. "Watch it!" another staff member called to him over my shoulder as we were speaking. "You know you aren't allowed to discuss those kinds of things!"

Perplexed, I turned to ask about his comment but he was already herding people out of the meeting room into another conference room for the union meeting. I asked if I could attend the union meeting and met with a polite refusal. Over the course of the next few weeks, I learned that the national health employees' union, SUTSAS (Syndicat autonome des travailleurs de la santé et de l'action sociale) was in the midst of an information boycott. In an attempt to leverage more bargaining power with the state, the union was refusing to submit any information to the district, the medical region, or the national offices of the health ministry. Daily activity logs, reasons for patient consultations, vaccination rates, and prescriptions given to patients were all included in the boycott.

Over the following twelve months as I established rapport with several of the head nurses by visiting them at their health posts and occasionally in their homes, I found that they largely regarded me as harmless and didn't view our conversations as a violation of the boycott. Although the union position was that information should not be reported to higher administrative units, in practice the boycott meant that most medical staff simply stopped keeping any records at all. There are no usable health data available for the Saint Louis medical district for the eighteen-month period of my research, or for the period immediately prior to and immediately after my study ended. Nonetheless, we can piece together a sense of Senegal's disease profile from published sources.

Numbers tell their own epidemiological story, but it is one that can be as partial and incomplete as the stories that come from the voices and experiences of everyday people. In the introduction to Senegal's *Annuaire Statistique* for 2005 (published in July 2006), the authors note that the data are incomplete, largely due to periodic union calls to boycott reporting procedures. In 2005 Senegal's total population was estimated to be slightly over 11 million people, and Senegal currently ranks 156 out of the 177 countries ranked on the Human Development Index. Just over 50 percent of Senegal's households are considered to be living below the poverty line, and 26 percent of the population lives on less than US $1 per day. Though I am quite familiar with the stark poverty and sense of crisis among Senegal's poor, particularly those living in rural areas, it is still striking that the millions of dollars spent on social and economic development have not translated into higher indicators, even when compared with other developing countries.

As in most developing countries, the primary health challenges in Senegal are infant and child mortality, maternal mortality, and the high rates of mortality and morbidity from endemic infectious diseases, particularly malaria and respiratory infections. The average life expectancy at birth in Senegal is 62 years (Population Reference Bureau 2007). Senegal is slightly below the global average life expectancy, which is 68 years (77 years for the more developed countries and 55 years for the least developed countries) (Population Reference Bureau 2008). Senegal's life expectancy compares favorably to the rest of sub-Saharan Africa, where average life expectancy is only 50 years. Maternal mortality ratios are notoriously high in sub-Saharan Africa, with an average of 900 maternal deaths per 100,000 births in 2005 (Population Reference Bureau 2008). Senegal's current ratio is below this average, but still exceedingly high at 401 (or 690 if one accepts the WHO's adjusted data). In the "most developed countries" (i.e., the North), maternal mortality ratios average around 10 deaths per 100,000 births, while in Latin America and the Caribbean they average 130 (Population Reference Bureau 2008).

Following the classic pattern of health transition, increasing rates of cancer, heart disease, hypertension, and diabetes are beginning to burden Senegal's health system, which is still overwhelmed by the usual diseases of poverty (cholera, diarrheal diseases, malaria, measles, malnutrition). In addition to the strain created by trying to prevent and treat both kinds of diseases, the distribution of resources within the health system is quite uneven. Throughout the 1990s the capital city of Dakar, which comprised 22 percent of Senegal's total population, received 40 percent of the total health budget (Ndiaye et al. 1997). Urban hospitals, particularly the teaching hospitals in Dakar, often have cutting-edge technology and surgical options for newer diseases while hospitals and clinics in outlying regions struggle to respond to cholera outbreaks and the spike in illness during the rainy season. Although it receives lots of donor funding, including money from the Global Fund for malaria and HIV/AIDS projects, the government spends only US $12 per person on health care per year.

Most of Senegal's health development aid over the past three decades has been directed at interventions for child survival and maternal health. These include programs to combat malnutrition, to increase vaccine coverage, campaigns for oral rehydration therapy, family planning campaigns, the promotion of prenatal visits, and attempts to increase the number of births attended by state-trained midwives or community birth attendants. In spite of millions of dollars spent on these initiatives by the United States Agency for International Development (USAID), among other donors, progress has been slow. Senegal's under-five mortality rate is perhaps the largest success; it decreased from

211 deaths per 1,000 children in 1986 to 143 per 1,000 in 2005. Nonetheless, according to estimates in 2005, only 10 percent of infants and children suffering from malnutrition received any medical care (Ministère de la Santé 2006).

Senegal's population is currently increasing at a rate of 3 percent per year (Population Reference Bureau 2008). Donors and government officials remain concerned about Senegal's population growth, in spite of the Cairo platform that emerged during the 1994 United Nations International Conference on Population and Development. This platform stresses women's and men's reproductive rights and voluntary decisions about contraception, and represented a step away from population control programs with demographic targets. In the wake of extremely well funded programs, Senegal's contraception prevalence rate (CPR) has increased from 4.8 percent in the early 1990s to 14 percent in 2005, but the total fertility rate (TFR) remains high at 5.3 (Ndiaye et al. 1992/93; Ministère de la Santé 2005). The percentage of women attended during childbirth by a trained health professional, 51 percent, has changed little since the early 1990s (see Table 4.1).[1]

These aggregate statistics provide a sense of Senegal's overall health status and change over the past thirty years, and national data allow for comparisons between countries. Senegal compares positively to many of its neighbors and other countries in sub-Saharan Africa to be sure, but these countries make up the bottom tier of the Health Development Index. Aggregate data also disguise the large variations in disease burdens among the rich and the poor, which to

TABLE 4.1

Senegal Health Data, 1986–2005

	Birth rate	Death rate	Maternal mortality ratio (Reported/ adjusted)	Under-five mortality	Contraception prevalence rate (CPR)	Total fertility rate (TFR)	% of Births attended
2005	36	10	401/690	143	14	5.3	51
1997	39	11	560	139	12.9	5.7	47
1992/93	40.8	12	510	157	4.8	6.0	47
1986	45.7	17	460	211		6.4	41

Sources: Foote et al. 1993; Ndiaye et al. 1986; Ndiaye et al. 1992/93; Ndiaye et al. 1997; Ministère de la Santé 2006; Population Reference Bureau 2007 and 2008; UN 1989; World Bank 2007.

some extent dovetail with the health gap between urban and rural areas. When the under-five mortality rate is disaggregated by income, the rate for the richest fifth of the population falls to 70 deaths per 1,000 children, while the rate for the poorest fifth is 181 per 1,000. Similarly, the total fertility rate for the poorest women is 7.4 while for those in the richest fifth it is 3.6. For women receiving care during childbirth, the rate among the poorest women drops to 20 percent (Population Reference Bureau 2007).

The health statistics for the Saint Louis region indicate that it is well below national averages on most counts, mainly because it is plagued with being largely rural and extremely poor. Although these data are incomplete (75 percent of the health reports were submitted for the region in 2005), one can identify important trends that help delineate the disease burden for children and adults. The first handicap facing Saint Louis residents is the relative lack of health infrastructure compared to other regions. There is one health post for every 16,406 residents of the region, while the national average is 1:11,874 (Ministère de la Santé 2006). Reproductive health indicators are similar: fewer than 50 percent of pregnant women in the region receive prenatal care, and only 9 percent of births are attended by a provider. While around 12 percent of married women in Senegal use some form of contraception, only 3 percent of women in the Saint Louis region do. These health disparities between residents of the Saint Louis region and the rest of the country are evident historically as well as in the most recent data sets. In the 1992 Demographic Health Survey, the infant mortality rate was 68:1000 nationally, but 108:1000 for the Northeast region where Saint Louis is located. Similarly, while the under-five mortality rate was 68:1000 for the country, the Northeast's rate was 83.7:1000 (Ndiaye et al. 1992/93).

One domain in which Senegal does appear to be doing extremely well is in the arena of HIV/AIDS prevention and treatment. The current estimates are that Senegal's overall seroprevalence rate is 0.7 percent, and the rate among women is 2.25 percent (Ministère de la Santé 2006). The epidemic remains concentrated among sex workers and men who have sex with men (MSM); rates may be as high as 15 to 20 percent among these vulnerable populations. There are numerous theories about why Senegal has been so successful at keeping its HIV rate low. In the 1980s the Senegalese government was one of the first African governments to acknowledge the pandemic and to begin aggressive education campaigns and blood screening. Senegal's system for regulating sex work, which dates back to the colonial period, provided a means of offering prevention education, HIV screening, and eventually treatment and support services to HIV positive sex workers.

Recognizing the importance of religious sanction for HIV/AIDS prevention and treatment activities, the government collaborated early on with Muslim and Catholic leaders to coordinate a unified approach to stopping AIDS. JAMRA and SIDA Service, Muslim and Catholic organizations, respectively, have been at the forefront of Senegal's dynamic civil society response to AIDS. Senegal has also received a tremendous amount of donor support from the Global Fund for AIDS, Malaria, and Tuberculosis. The increasing ability of the NGO sector to enforce accountability and good governance of these funds has also had a tremendous effect on Senegal's success (Jurgens and Dia 2006). The government has made a financial commitment to universal access to antiretroviral medication, and these medications are offered free of charge. Health professionals and activists still warn against complacency, particularly since the relatively low rates of HIV in neighboring countries suggest that Senegal's prevention strategies have not truly been tested yet (Engelberg 2005).

The Saint Louis Medical District: People and Places

The medical district of Saint Louis is one of forty-five such districts in the country; districts are the smallest administrative units of the public health sector. The district consists of fourteen community clinics referred to as dispensaries or *postes de santé*. Ten of these clinics are located in Saint Louis proper, one in each of the main neighborhoods. The remaining four clinics are considered rural or peri-urban as they serve rural communities surrounding Saint Louis. The health post in Tassinère, situated about 18 kilometers outside of Saint Louis, serves villages in the Ganjool region. The head nurses at the rural clinics supervise the village health huts in their zones. The health huts represent the lowest level of biomedical care available to Senegalese living in rural areas. The health hut workers, who are mainly women, are trained in first aid and in the treatment of common illnesses such as malaria and childhood diarrhea. In addition to these activities, the health hut workers are first and foremost birth attendants.

The personnel and activities at rural and urban health posts are very similar, save for the prevalence of maternity wards at the rural dispensaries. At the head of each health post is the *infirmier-chef de poste* (ICP). All ICPs have graduated from the government nursing school and have received the diploma *infirmier d'état*. The ICPs oversee a staff of as many as ten people, from the cashier, who sells the consultation tickets and often the pharmaceuticals, to the midwives who are assisted by birth attendants. There are typically three to four nurses' aides and community health workers who do first-aid procedures, help with vaccinations, and generally assist the nurses and midwives.

According to the health reforms passed in the early 1990s, the ICP should collaborate with the neighborhood health committee to identify strategic goals for the health post and to manage the profits from the sale of consultation tickets and pharmaceuticals. Health committees are comprised of elected officers (president, vice president, treasurer, and secretary) who represent the neighborhood and serve as the liaison between community members and the health system. They are charged with sponsoring activities and education addressing the eight tenets of primary health care, and assisting to identify and resolve community health problems.[2] The committee ideally articulates neighborhood health needs to the ICP, mobilizes local resources to address these problems, carries out health activities, improves the dispensary through restoration or the purchasing of additional equipment, and evaluates these ongoing activities to correct problems and identify new short-term goals. Last but not least, the committees are responsible for setting the correct prices for consultation tickets and pharmaceuticals, finding other means of generating revenue for the clinic, and managing all of the funds earned by clinic activities.

The highest administrative tier of the medical district consists of the chief medical doctor (*médecin-chef de district*, or MC), whom I will refer to as Dr. Faal, and the district supervisors. At the time of my research there were five supervisors in the district whose areas of responsibility were primary health care, vaccinations, maternal and child health and family planning, social work, and health education. Supervisors work with Dr. Faal to coordinate in-service training sessions for the technical staff and on annual planning for the district. They help him facilitate the monthly coordination meetings during which the supervisory team meets with the ICPs and midwives from each clinic. Every other month they hold "large group meetings" to which a representative from each dispensary's health committee is invited to attend. The supervision team periodically visits each post to review their books, to control their stock of medicine, and to conduct evaluations.

The MC oversees all district activities and is ultimately responsible for the quality of service and care provided by the dispensaries under his supervision. He supervises the approximately fifty district staff members, including the fourteen ICPs, the ten district midwives, thirteen community health aides and thirteen nurses' aides, and the remaining miscellaneous personnel. As he was the only medical doctor working for the district, Dr. Faal received patients several mornings a week. He spent much of the rest of his time attending regional and local-level meetings, overseeing the supervisory staff, and coordinating the district's monthly meetings.

Decentralization, Community Management, and User Fees in Saint Louis

Three elements of change have been central to the restructuring of Senegal's health system: decentralization, the formalization of "community participation" via health committees, and user fees. Most of these reforms are the result of many years of experimentation. From the mid-1970s to the present, the Senegalese government has tried to reconcile a primary health care strategy that promotes accessibility, equity, and quality of care with the state's limited ability to fund the health system. The external shock of austerity programs from the 1980s forward provided additional incentive to embark on significant reforms to the health system. During the 1980s and 1990s, ongoing experiments with community management and voluntary user fees evolved into a partially privatized system, in which user fees and drug sales finance a significant portion of each health structure's operating costs.

The state continues to subsidize significant portions of the public sector, but in the newly decentralized system these funds flow through local and regional channels instead of directly from the Ministry of Health to the medical districts. The government has also delegated certain responsibilities to local governments and recommended that 9 percent of their budgets (from local taxes and revenues) be spent on the health sector. Decentralization has brought much confusion to local government and administration. Difficulties stem from complications such as general misunderstanding and ignorance of the new laws by local officials, lack of institutional capacity, and the lack of resources to supplement greatly reduced state spending.

Decentralization and City Politics in Saint Louis

Decentralization is designed to make the state more responsive and adaptable to local and regional needs, thereby strengthening democracy by increasing the accountability of elected officials to their constituents (Derman et al. 2000; Spierenberg et al. 1999; Webster 1992). In Senegal, the mandate of local government is to "ensure, for the entirety of its constituent population, the highest possible quality of life" (Article 88, Code des Collectivités locales). An ongoing struggle between the medical administrators and the city officials was the most visible sign of the pains associated with decentralization. The most prominent battle was about water and electricity at the district's urban dispensaries. During my research the majority of the city's ten dispensaries, the lowest level of care in the health system, were without water and electricity. According to the MC, when the national government stopped paying utilities at local health facilities and delegated this task to city governments, Saint Louis' administration refused to take over the expense.

At the district's staff meetings, the monthly update from each city dispensary turned into a ritual of reminding the medical chief that they were expected to provide adequate, hygienic care without the benefits of water or electricity. Every month the nurse from Ndar-Tuut would remind Dr. Faal that her clinic had gone over a year without water. Another nurse would note that he hoped his water problem would be resolved soon because his staff were tired of walking around the neighborhood every morning asking housewives to donate water to the health post. Every month the medical chief replied that he was still negotiating with the city. Some of the more financially successful health posts decided to pay the utility bills with their own revenues. For the health posts in the poorest neighborhoods this was out of the question.

Dr. Faal spent months trying to resolve the utility problem. After many missed appointments, the mayor's secretary-general finally attended a district staff meeting in September. One of the district administrators welcomed him to the meeting and explained that as many of the city's dispensaries had been without water and electricity for over two years, the medical district wanted an update on how the mayor was proposing to resolve the issue. "Well, the state imposed decentralization on us. The water company, the electric company, they now sell privately and they treat the mayor's office like any other client. If the bills are not paid they cut off service. We are negotiating on past-due bills." He added that when the city government first became responsible for utilities, it urged the medical district to reduce its use of water, but the bills kept getting more expensive. "Decentralization has not been easy," he argued. "It has meant a transfer of responsibility [to the city] with no transfer of means."

The mayor's representative explained the compromise he hoped to make with the medical district. Since they still received a US $1,000 subsidy from the national government, they would put this sum toward the medical district's utilities, but the district would need to pay for all utilities above that sum. One of the district supervisors objected to this suggestion, "But that money comes from the national government. What about the 9 percent of its budget that the city is supposed to spend on health?" Another nurse joined the protest, "We haven't received any pharmaceuticals from the city! Where has all the money allocated for drugs gone?" The city official tried to respond to these complaints, but he confessed that the city had few options. "We do not have many resources. We have no big factories, no local industry, no major commerce here. We just don't have the ability to give any more support to the medical district." This deflection of responsibility provoked outrage from the medical staff. The midwife from the Lodo dispensary confronted the official, "I can't believe the city is saying it won't take responsibility for the health of the population! You are saying you don't have the resources, but you have some, so it is a question of priorities. You were supposed to replace the state. If you abandon us it is going to be a total catastrophe!"

Mr. Turpin acknowledged that the city would like to do more, but for an undetermined period of time it would be unable to pay for the clinics' water and electricity. The secretary-general was correct about the city's shortage of resources. A UNESCO study highlights that the city of Saint Louis spends 80 percent of its total budget on personnel (Spierenberg et al. 1999, 7). Therefore, 1 percent of the city's population, the city employees, consumes 80 percent of its resources. With no resolution in sight coming from the city, several health committees decided they would attempt to pay for their own water and electricity using health post profits. Others continued to wait it out, and medical personnel carried on working under less than ideal conditions.

In addition to a lack of financial resources, Saint Louis has experienced other problems associated with decentralization. While the country was well into the implementation of decentralized management of the health system, no rural council had yet created a health development plan. Most elected officials (81 percent of those surveyed) were unaware that such plans should exist for every district and were to be executed jointly by health administrators and local government. Other officials (60 percent) believed there is no restriction on how they spend their state budgets, in spite of funds being earmarked for particular sectors (Ministère de l'Economie, des Finances, et du Plan 1998, 46). Nurses from rural clinics often complained that their rural council had approved the year's budget without designating any funds for the health sector. These nurses felt they were intentionally excluded from budget meetings and that they had no leverage to obtain the cooperation of rural officials.

The process of decentralization has been challenging due to constrained resources, but also because most local officials are unfamiliar with the texts on decentralization and do not understand their new responsibilities. Most have never received any kind of training on how decentralization should work at local and regional levels. As a result, a significant portion of elected officials feel it is not their responsibility to respond to community health concerns and problems, but the responsibility of the neighborhood health committees and medical personnel. Meanwhile, medical district staff argue that local government should be proactive in the creation and implementation of a community health agenda. There is dire lack of planning and management, exacerbated by weak institutional capacity and few resources that can be allocated to handle the increasing number of responsibilities. Health care personnel have borne the brunt of decentralization; they have been cut loose by the state, and their concerns and problems have not been assumed by regional and district officials.

In the years since decentralization, the municipality of Saint Louis has shown little capacity to respond to community needs or to "ensure the highest quality of life for all." Decentralization has not strengthened local democratic processes, but instead has left public officials and civil servants frustrated and in a deadlock with one another. While these two components of the public sector are attempting to negotiate a working relationship and a consensus on their respective roles and responsibilities, the general population has largely been excluded from this deliberative process. In particular, women are poorly represented in local government and have been absent from these conversations. Statistics for the region of Saint Louis suggest that women account for only 20 percent of municipality officials and rural council members, and they are also poorly represented on the neighborhood health committees.

The Perils of Participatory Management

"But Dr. Faal," the nurse protested, "what do I do about this health committee president? He has refused to step down for two terms now, and everyone knows he is no good. Our general assembly is coming up and I have no way to get him to step down." This was a frequent lament at the spring staff meetings as health committee election time rolled around. Many health posts had dysfunctional health committees, and nurses knew that if they could not facilitate a transition in health committee membership they would be stuck for another two years. Dr. Faal's response was consistent from meeting to meeting, "The code regarding health committees has not changed since 1992. The maximum term for any committee member is two terms of two years. You are the ICP, the person in charge of the health post. It is up to you to enforce the new codes and texts. You simply tell him that after having served two terms he is no longer eligible to be a candidate for the committee." Although Dr. Faal and his district supervisors repeatedly stressed that the "codes and texts" governing health structures were clear, medical personnel continuously confronted the enormous slippage between law and practice in the daily operations of their health posts.

Senegal began experimenting with health committees (formerly called Health Promotion Associations) in the early 1970s, but they were not given full legal recognition until 1992. General assemblies are organized by neighborhood every two years to elect the committee members. To participate in a general assembly one must be a member of a registered women's group, a neighborhood association, or a sporting and cultural association. The Ministry of Health has recognized that these committees need to be independent of political, social, religious, and ethnic factions, but since their inception they have been plagued by a number of problems.

Early evaluations of the health committees conducted in the mid-1990s revealed several challenges. Health committees were rapidly politicized and became closely tied to political parties; being elected an officer of a health committee was actually more like a political appointment that would ensure the appointee easy access to large amounts of cash (Lo et al. 1997). The discretionary power of the committees over clinic funds made leadership positions very attractive; the officers tended to be retirees, unemployed politicians, and local notables. Committees were not reelected every two years as dictated by the texts, nor were they representative of the population as a whole. Meanwhile, the medical personnel felt completely excluded from financial planning and management and were resentful of the committees for misusing the funds that had been earned through their own hard work (Lo et al. 1997).

In spite of the Ministry of Health's attempt to respond to these initial evaluations, newspaper headlines in the late 1990s continued to decry scandal after scandal, as thousands and thousands of dollars in cash and pharmaceuticals went missing from one health structure or another. Participatory management of health facilities is in and of itself a complex endeavor, and the stakes changed significantly in 1997 when Senegal's decentralization laws (passed in 1996) were implemented. Medical personnel experienced this transition as a dramatic shrinking of resources for the health sector, but more importantly, each health post had to rely mainly on its own profits to ensure a constant supply of pharmaceuticals and to pay for overhead expenses. With so much riding on the financial resources of each health post, oversight and control of health post profits became the central point of tension between the head nurses and the health committees.

At every monthly staff meeting, when the head nurses provided an update of their health post's activities, the complaints about the misdeeds of the health committees began again. "We had our health committee election but the same president was reelected," groaned the nurse from Get Ndar. From the Bango midwife: "We have scheduled our election but the president refuses to step down." Other conflicts emerged when health committees refused to disburse funds for items that the head nurse needed. At the July meeting, when both district staff and health committee members were in attendance, a head nurse confronted his health committee treasurer for refusing to grant him his US $2 transport stipend for the day's meeting. "Well," the treasurer responded, "we gave it to him last month, and then we found out that he didn't attend the meeting. This month we thought we would wait to see if he actually showed up." This admission provoked immediate reaction from the medical personnel who countered that it was not the job of the health committees to supervise them. Dr. Faal, as usual, tried to mediate between the nurses and the health committee members by clarifying the rules and procedures concerning spending.

In April the district supervisors held a meeting with newly elected health committee presidents and treasurers to hear their concerns and to field questions about health post operations. I learned about it with the rest of the medical personnel at the April staff meeting. Jallo, the social work supervisor, launched into his report of the meeting with a cautionary tone: "They came here to hold court. They ranted and raved against the head nurses. We must be very vigilant with them—they are dangerous. The slightest thing and they will go off." Most of the medical personnel were not even aware that this meeting had taken place. Tensions rose in the room as they claimed they had been denounced by the health committees in a secret meeting where they were unable to defend themselves. The primary health care supervisor tried to diffuse the mounting anger, "Look, they are our partners. We have to work with them. We have to accept that the population now has a say in government health services. We have to accept their role in managing these services."

This incident touched off a lengthy and animated debate about the ongoing difficulties with the health committees. While there were some specific allegations, like health committees not wanting to spend money on items like cotton balls and iodine that could not be resold, the main difficulty was the sense that nurses and medical aides were being micromanaged by the health committees. This frustration emerged in a historical moment in which the power, status, and authority of medical personnel had declined significantly. They were angered to find themselves having to answer to lay members of the community, many of whom are illiterate and have never attended school. Some nurses were willing to accept their own transgressions; one angry head nurse acknowledged, "I admit it, I have never paid for pharmaceuticals. He who works at the hotel eats at the hotel!" Yet the majority felt that if their own work ethic and management practice was somewhat loose, the health committees are far worse. As the nurse from Jaamagenn asserted, "If they accuse us of theft, it is the pot calling the kettle black! They are the ones who are stealing and everyone knows it. They bring everyone they know and claim they have indigent status and should get free treatment." This set off a storm of follow-up accusations that the health committees are impossible to control. One nurse summed up their feelings by declaring, "If they want war, we'll make war!"

After the initial squall of protest, Dr. Faal addressed the numerous concerns voiced by his staff. The supervisory team had investigated several of the claims made by the health committees. While some were greatly exaggerated, others were well founded. In Dr. Faal's words, "Every month we ask you for updates and you say you have no major news. You can't say this in a meeting when in fact your health post is nearly bankrupt. The health committees brought some bad practices to light, and it is your responsibility to keep the health post running well." As the medical personnel became less defensive, the supervisors encouraged them to rethink their partnerships with the committees. Many of the nurses agreed that in the past they had ignored or dismissed the health committees, and that under the new system this was no longer possible. The medical personnel have had to come to terms with the reality that, "if we leave the committees alone, they will eat all the money," and that the committees are also eager to disclose any wrongdoings they observe on the part of medical staff. While many of the personnel lodged bitter complaints about the injustice of this situation, most acknowledged that it was in the interest of all to establish a good relationship with the health committees.

By the end of the April staff meeting, the medical personnel seemed resigned to the necessity of collaborating with the health committees, but the health committees continued to suspect health post staff of wrongdoing. In June 1999 Dr. Faal organized a training to orient the new health committee members and to facilitate a better working relationship with the medical staff. As part of the orientation, Dr. Faal provided an overview of the basic operations of the health posts, the management tools, and the process for annual monitoring and evaluation of each health post's performance. The committee members were very keen on the idea of monitoring, as Dr. Faal stressed that annual evaluations allowed both medical personnel and community members to assess the quality of care at each health structure and to develop action plans for improvement.

In the midst of their questions about this process, Dr. Faal had to admit that the district had not been able to conduct monitoring since 1996 because of the health worker (SUTSAS) strike.[3] The health committee members seized upon this as irrefutable evidence that the union's objective was to avoid being supervised by either the health committees or their district administrators. "We must find a way to do monitoring," one committee member asserted, "as that is the way to reveal all of the misdoings of the personnel." Although Dr. Faal and the district supervisors eventually steered the discussions back to the training agenda, learning of the information boycott provided many health committee members with sufficient evidence that they should take matters into their own hands.

The contentious relationships between health committee members and the district's medical personnel continued throughout my field research. Though Dr. Faal and his administrative staff attempted to resolve the frequent disputes and insisted upon following all of the designated management protocols, both health committees and medical staff found ways around the regulations. The president of Get Ndar told me that his health committee keeps a large sum of petty cash on hand so they will not have to secure the permission of the head nurse before making purchases. He also said they give the medical staff generous bonuses to "keep them in line." Medical personnel, too, had their own strategies, such as showing up late for work and taking full advantage of their access to free pharmaceuticals. Vieux Mamadu Seck, a political outsider who was elected treasurer of the Pikine health committee in 1999, summed up many people's feelings about participatory management of the health posts: "The health committees and the health post staff are like two dogs facing off over a piece of meat. Neither side is trustworthy."

The Senegalese Ministry of Health has touted the need for participatory approaches to health for over two decades. The unveiling of the government's five-year health plan in 1999 came with the declaration that there must be a "full partnership" between the state and the population to assure the highest quality of health care. Nonetheless, a debilitating atmosphere of mistrust and antagonism existed between the Saint Louis health committees and their "partners in health," the clinic medical staff. These ongoing problems correspond with prevailing critiques of decentralization and increasing the responsibilities of local bodies, that is, that these processes often work to strengthen prevailing inequalities (Turshen 1999).

The importance of trust in the functioning of health systems and in medical encounters is receiving renewed attention in the literature on health reform. Bloom and colleagues assert that trust is a fundamental component of the social contract revolving around medical care (Bloom et al. 2008). To understand how health systems work, and for them to function more effectively, scholars and policymakers must understand the mechanisms by which trust is generated through encounters between patients and providers and through "socially legitimate regulatory regimes" (Bloom et al. 2008, 2077). In the best-case scenario, government and citizenry share expectations of the health system and how it will be evaluated. Brazil offers an innovative approach in which an ongoing, participatory, deliberative process of health planning was carried out by organizing annual large public meetings where citizens, civil society, and government debated about the priorities and future directions of Brazil's health system. This process facilitated a national consensus on the government's role as guarantor of public health (Cornwall and Shankland 2008). In the Senegalese case, the health committees are designed to serve as the vehicle through which state and civil society collaborate on agenda setting, problem solving, and improving the delivery of health services. The high level of mistrust between medical personnel and the health committee members points to a shaky foundation for a social contract regarding health, in spite of the government's continued commitment to "participatory" management of the health sector.

Beyond the conflicts between health committees and medical personnel at the district health posts, the election of health committee officers was quite partisan, and general assemblies and elections occurred infrequently. Vieux Mamadu Seck explained that the same core group of men dominates all aspects of local civil society and local government.[4] He comments: "Wherever you go, you see the same handful of old men running things. Whether it is the health committee, the school board, the summer soccer league, neighborhood development associations, or local political party meetings, it's the same guys everywhere you go." Decentralization and community management of health facilities have provided new opportunities for local elites to gain access to political power and material resources.

The principles of participatory management are the basis of the health committees, but the general assemblies exclude a broad base of potential stakeholders who have important knowledge about community health needs. In the training sessions for newly elected officers who would serve on the health committees from spring 1999 to spring 2001, not a single woman was in the group. The demographics of these officers were nearly identical to the local council members and members of local government. The health committee representatives were all male, and almost all were over age fifty. Not surprisingly, it's the same group of men described by Vieux Seck who sit on school committees, head neighborhood associations, dominate local politics, and benefit from the social and material capital inherent in these positions. This politicization of health committees, and the ways these positions can be used for personal gain, has also worked to erode trust in participatory management of health structures.

User Fees and Quality of Care

Most residents of Saint Louis have very little understanding of how the government health system has been affected by decentralization or the institutionalization of health committees. The subject of user fees, on the other hand, elicited endless stories about the difficulty of seeking medical care at city health posts. Two main problems surfaced in conversations about user fees and privatization: biomedical care was either too expensive to use at all, or the quality of services at neighborhood health posts was so poor that Saint Louis residents were unwilling to pay for it. Each of these complaints creates dilemmas for patients who often borrow to pay for medical services and embark on elaborate medical itineraries to find the nurses and health posts that are worth their time and money.

Clinic gates are the place where most Saint Louis residents encounter privatization. Patients pay a consultation fee in order to pass through the gates and wait in line for a consultation. In the late 1990s consultation fees were US 50 cents at health posts, and US $10 at the Saint Louis hospital. The cost of consultation tickets loomed large in the minds of Saint Lousiens when they reflected on recent changes to the health system. Kumba Gey, a Pikine resident, explained: "These days, if you are ill, if you can't pay for the ticket, anything might happen to you. If you can't pay for the prescription or the procedure, they won't even touch you." Although the user fees at neighborhood health posts were quite modest, even for the urban poor, the limited package of services available at health posts meant that many patients were quickly referred to higher, more expensive levels of care. This is the fragmentation of health services that Janes describes in settings where market-based health reforms have been carried out (Janes 2004).

At the neighborhood health posts "buying a ticket" is usually followed by standing or sitting in a crowded waiting room for several hours. After this wait, one sees a distracted nurse or midwife who scribbles out a prescription after three or four minutes of consultation. As Faama Faal comments, "You can go to the clinic and they don't even examine you. They just ask you 'what's wrong' or 'what's wrong with your child?' and then they write you a prescription and send you off to buy it." The patient goes to the clinic dispensary to get the prescription filled, assuming the clinic has pharmaceuticals in stock. The availability of drugs is one of the most significant benefits of the Bamako Initiative in Senegal; most clinics now have pharmaceuticals in stock for those who can afford them.

Mothers and grandmothers, as household caretakers, feel the effects of privatization acutely as they typically accompany the patient and interact with medical personnel. They often borrow cash or solicit donations at the hospital gates to secure the consultation fee that is demanded before any service will be rendered. Much preventative and curative medicine is sought outside of the biomedical sphere, yet Saint Louis residents recognize that receiving adequate biomedical care in a timely manner is often a matter of life and death in cases of grave illness. Biomedicine is certainly not the exclusive option for managing illness, but it is an option that is valued and desired by most people and is seen as the most appropriate method for treatment of malaria, hypertension, diabetes, and complications with childbirth, among others.

During focus group discussions, women recounted stories of prolonged illnesses that occurred as a result of an inability to pay for care. When asked about the difficulties accessing care in the privatized health system, Pikine resident Salimata So explains: "At the hospital they will actually examine you, they actually look at your body and follow-up on your treatment. But you have to have money. If you don't have money, you can't get medical care. No money, no care." Other Pikine residents echoed this sense that money was an important consideration in therapeutic decisions. Not only do patients pay the consultation fees, but in the resource-constrained environment of the health system they also leveraged better care from providers by paying them directly. Another focus group participant elaborated on these realities: "Every single door, money is what opens it. If you bribe the hospital staff they will take care of you morning, noon, and night. But if you don't have money, you lie there and they walk right past you." In other interviews women described sharing daily meals and tea with hospital staff, particularly janitors, so that their hospitalized family member would have access to clean bathrooms and would receive regular cleaning services in their hospital rooms.

Although the Bamako Initiative has solved problems with the availability of essential medicines, Pikine resident Khadi Jaagn illustrates lingering frustrations with the unpredictable services at city health posts: "Sometimes you are ill and you go to the dispensary but it's closed, and you don't have enough money to go to the hospital, and even if you have enough money to go to the hospital they write you a prescription that you can't afford. Or you go to the hospital and there is no doctor there. Our clinic here in Pikine, it's hard enough to go and find it open, or you want to vaccinate your child and they tell you there aren't any vaccines." Khadi's observations coincide with the well-known complaints that many health committees lodged against the nurses and midwives and the quality of the health system in general. The medical staff work irregular hours, there are frequent vaccine shortages, and for many poor residents of Saint Louis even generic pharmaceuticals are too expensive.

Hospital visits require more patience and more cash. At the hospital, patients pay their consultation fee and then pay for every subsequent medical procedure, from the insertion of IVs to the administration of necessary drugs. By the time most patients arrive at the hospital they are gravely ill or near death and require several immediate interventions. The delivery of life-saving drugs is often delayed while a family member is sent to the hospital pharmacy to purchase medication. If the prescribed drug is not available at the hospital pharmacy, a family member will make the rounds of the private pharmacies in town hoping to find the pharmaceutical in time to save the patient.

The pronounced emphasis on fees for services created tremendous amounts of skepticism about the motivations of health post nurses and hospital staff. One focus group participant asserted: "They [health care workers] don't even care that this person is a human being like them. They are only worrying about their money, they aren't worrying about the lives of the patients." Saint Louis residents were rightly concerned about the costs of care, but these concerns were compounded by their perception that the quality of care at government health facilities had declined in recent years, and was quite uneven from clinic to clinic. When patients confront the impersonal nature of the privatized system, they often conclude that doctors and nurses are only interested in extracting user fees, not in saving lives.

Nurses and other medical personnel often told me that they too are frustrated by the need to demand money for health care, and they have a difficult time playing the dual role of service provider and fee collector. There was widespread consensus among nurses in Saint Louis that many of the recent reforms had been poorly executed and were not adequately explained to the population. The most senior professionals reminisced about how health care workers, especially doctors and nurses, were once among the most respected government employees. Now they are often seen as the embodiment of everything that is wrong with the health care system. They are also severely underpaid, so those who remain in the public sector often turn to strategies like selling prescriptions under the table or running parallel clinics within public health care facilities. Their dilemmas and challenges become apparent when we take a closer look at the near-collapse of the Pikine health post in chapter 5.

Tallying the Balance Sheet: Decentralization and Health Reform

The collapse of African health systems is often quickly dismissed as the negative result of structural adjustment lending and the rise of market-based policies. "Neoliberalism" has become a throwaway label to describe these trends, but it cannot capture the qualitative shifts taking place as governments radically reshape the structure, organization, and financial underpinnings of their health systems. The Bamako Initiative institutionalized community financing of the health system through user fees and a generic drug plan, but it was health sector decentralization that most significantly affected day-to-day operations of health posts and medical clinics. The convergence of decentralization and health reform produced multilayered conflicts in Saint Louis. These tensions are most evident in the struggles between the medical district and the city government, and between medical professionals and community leaders.

The Bamako Initiative was an attempt to implement efficiency-driven reforms with a utilitarian objective, to provide a minimum level of care to the greatest number of citizens in the face of shrinking state resources. Little attention was given to whether these reforms would produce equitable outcomes or improve access to care for the poorest and most marginal populations. User fee exemptions and safety net provisions have proven cumbersome and inadequate, thereby leaving many people completely outside of the government system (Ridde 2003). The uneven quality of services at PHC clinics contributes to a patchwork or fragmented system in which Saint Louis residents make strategic decisions about when and where to seek medical care to stretch their limited health resources. These kinds of reforms create "poor medicine for poor people" as the scope and quality of primary care declines and people are left to fend for themselves in the private sector (Janes 2003, 2004).

Paralleling this partial privatization of the health system, government rhetoric about "responsibilization" and "state-citizen partnerships" draws attention to the obligations of individual citizens to take charge of their own health. Veiled in references to partnership and a participatory approach to health care, these idioms deflect attention from the structural inequalities that influence health status and access to medical care. They invoke liberal notions of "rights and responsibilities" of citizens and health consumers, yet Roberts and Reich (2002) remind us that the right to "take charge of one's health" is meaningless without adequate resources to do so. The current reform strategies fail to acknowledge the kinds of social, political, and material resources that are prerequisites to exercising these kinds of rights. At a minimum, residents of Saint Louis need cash to pay the consultation fees at city clinics, and the city government requires capital to invest in a primary health care strategy.

The sheer insufficiency of financial resources for the medical district itself was the backdrop against which the daily dramas between the health committees and the medical personnel played out. The transfer of financial responsibility for the medical district from the national government to the commune of Saint Louis has meant that the medical district is left with almost no resources aside from the small profits of its medical structures. In 1999 each health post received a donation of approximately US $800 of pharmaceuticals from the Ministry of Health. The district received funds from donors to organize training sessions and supervisory trips, but the donation of medicines was the only direct contribution to the medical structures themselves. The dispensaries were running on small profit margins, using them to pay for all of their overhead expenses. In the face of limited support from national and local government, some health posts continued to offer a minimum of services and access to generic pharmaceuticals while others continuously flirted with bankruptcy.

In addition to stressing cost-recovery and generic pharmaceuticals, the Bamako Initiative mandated the reorganization of daily operations at the health posts. As few people have actually studied the new codes and legal texts or been trained in their application, there remains a significant amount of slippage between these laws and their enactment in the district. Varying interpretations of these reforms create opportunities for disagreement and corruption. The greatest challenge for the nurses is collaborating with the health committees, particularly about financial decisions. Nurses are still responsible for the daily operations of the dispensaries, and both their superiors and the population at large hold them accountable. This accountability is an annoyance to some and it infuriates others, especially nurses whose health committees have been overly eager to monitor them. The committees are full of potential for mismanagement, and they are also thought to be dangerous and threatening because they can expose illegitimate practices on the part of the district personnel.

Although he was not able to resolve all of the district's problems during his tenure as medecin-chef, Dr. Faal remained optimistic about the potential of the reforms to overcome many of the constraints facing Senegal's health system.[5] He is a strong supporter of the Bamako Initiative and participatory management approaches; he claims that these reforms have produced the greatest results in rural areas where the population previously had almost no access to pharmaceuticals. Yet he concedes that the health committee elections are not run democratically, and that meaningful participation has not yet been achieved as committees are not representative of all stakeholders.

Women's near total exclusion from the jockeying taking place in the medical district raises important questions about the implementation of community-based management of the health sector, and the kind of social capital that might be necessary to participate in these structures. Although the procedures for health committee elections are designed to include traditionally weak constituencies, particularly women and youth, there is little evidence that these participatory approaches have surmounted existing hierarchies of age and gender. Janes's warning to scrutinize the "emergent social forms amidst declining state power and political decentralization" that are becoming the favored agents of participation is a timely reminder that civil society is not without its own inherent structural inequalities (2004, 463). Without concerted effort to address these inequalities, they will be reproduced in the new social and political spaces emerging under the rubric of "participation."

In spite of their marginalization from the health committees, women in Saint Louis are by no means passive in the face of disease. They voice discontent with the quality of services at their neighborhood dispensaries, and they often take their business to other neighborhood clinics or directly to the city hospital. As Bloom et al. (2008) emphasize, analysts of health systems must be careful to avoid assumptions that the urban and rural poor are incapable of making informed choices about where to seek medical care. Leonard's work in Tanzania demonstrates that poor households regularly make strategic decisions to frequent better providers and to bypass lower-quality ones (2007). In addition to choosing carefully among medical professionals working in the Saint Louis district, women rely on a network of service providers in the informal sector, especially lay midwives, for many of their health care needs. They are harsh in their evaluations of local biomedical care and they demonstrate resourcefulness in their daily struggles to manage family health problems. By making do on the margins of the formal health sector, women demonstrate their implicit critique of a health system that has failed to address their needs. Their health strategies are the focus of chapters 6 and 7.

5

Market-Based Medicine and Shantytown Politics in Pikine

My first trip to the Pikine health post gave me a good sense of how difficult it is for Pikine residents to seek care there. My research assistant and I set out from the main road on the sandy footpaths that wind their way through the congested neighborhood toward the Senegal River. Even for a lifelong Pikine resident it is easy to become disoriented in the heart of Pikine as small paths can suddenly dead-end on someone's doorstep, or the path you have chosen becomes so narrow and twisted that you can't tell if there will be a sudden turn ahead taking you in the wrong direction. After about twenty-five minutes of trudging through beach sand (and stopping several times to ask for directions), my research assistant and I made it to the doors of the clinic. It was late morning, and the central waiting area was filled with women and children sitting on benches, standing against the walls, and congregating near the entrance. The head nurse Abdu was busy seeing patients in a small clinic room, so we chatted with the ticket vendor and other auxiliary staff as we waited to greet him.

At first glance the health post seemed relatively ordinary. Most new construction in Saint Louis uses cement blocks and corrugated metal or plastic roofing, and the dispensary followed this model. I soon noticed that there were no lights, and the interior rooms appeared to be quite dim. After we joked with the staff about how difficult it was to find the clinic, they responded that their inaccessible location was the least of their problems. "Look here," said one of the nurses' aides, "do you see these marks?" She was pointing to some corrosion on the metal doorframes in the waiting area. "These are the water marks from the flooding. Every rainy season we get flooded out and have to shut down for a month or two." Our conversation continued through the litany of staff complaints about the health post as we waited. Eventually the nurse Abdu Joob appeared from the consultation room and greeted us warmly. He said he was pleased we had made it all the way out to his health post so we could see just how far away it is. He explained that he would love to talk with us and we should set up an interview for an evening that week. I agreed that we would come to his house at the designated time, and we headed back to the main road for lunch.

I had no idea at the time how fortunate we had been to find Abdu busy working at the dispensary on the day of our impromptu visit. According to Pikine residents, as much as half of the time they go, the health post is closed or he isn't there. Both Abdu and the Pikine health post had a dismal reputation among the city's health committee members. They were convinced that he was at the root of all of the management problems at the post. Just as backward Pikine was often the fodder for jokes from residents of other Saint Louis neighborhoods, the Pikine health post represented the worst medical facility in the district. At district staff meetings, Abdu and his support staff were often teased about their dispensary constantly being on the verge of collapse.

Chapter 4 illustrated how the Bamako Initiative and decentralization have affected the medical district's daily operations and health budget. This chapter provides a neighborhood-centered view of these processes from the perspectives of people living and working in Pikine. The Pikine dispensary offers a particularly dramatic case of the potential problems with health reform and decentralization. Yet nearly all of the difficulties that emerged in Pikine reflect widespread trends in countries undergoing market-based reforms, including declining access to care and deteriorating quality of care (Janes et al. 2006; Schoepf et al. 2000; Turshen 1999).

Some of the health post's problems stemmed from issues that confront Pikine as a whole: a large and growing population, acute poverty, and virtually no infrastructure. As one of the poorest neighborhoods in Saint Louis, Pikine was an unlikely candidate for cost-recovery via user fees and the sale of generic medicines. Few residents of Pikine know how to navigate the city's social services system to claim indigent status, which would entitle them to free medical care at city dispensaries. There are no accurate census data for Pikine, but my estimate is that a third of Pikine's households would easily qualify as indigent. In spite of the recognized need for safety nets for the poor who cannot afford to pay for care (Janes 2004), inequities have been exacerbated in Senegal's process of health reform.

The health post was also plagued by dysfunctions related to its personnel, which included Abdu, the head nurse, and Daba, the senior midwife. Both Abdu and Daba were frustrated about being employed at the "worst" health post located in the "worst" neighborhood in the city. In addition to the demoralized staff, Pikine had an uneven experience with community management. Like many other dispensaries in Saint Louis, the Pikine health post had several health committees that were incapable of sound management, while others outright embezzled funds. Each of these factors contributed to the deterioration of the health post's finances and staff morale. In February 1999 when a new health committee was elected, the health post had no pharmaceuticals in stock, no savings in its bank account, and it had incurred a large number of debts.

The story of the near-demise and gradual recovery of the Pikine health post demonstrates the complexity of implementing health reforms in a contentious social setting where different social actors jockey for power, influence, and access to material and pharmacological resources. Although Pikine's experience represents a worst-case scenario, it also illuminates the larger structural problems In the medical district, where health reforms have often worked to reinforce the power base of local elites while rendering medical care even less accessible to the urban poor.

"If you get sick in Pikine, you won't get well in Pikine."—Mamadu Seck

Vieux Mamadu Seck, a retired electric company employee in his sixties, was elected treasurer of the Pikine Health committee at the February general assembly.[1] By his own account he was more surprised at this turn of events than anyone else: "I never wanted to get involved with the health post because it had such a bad reputation. Personally, with my seventeen children, I am more interested in the school. But at the general assembly they wanted to list me as a candidate, and you know if people ask you to do something and you refuse, the next time you might need them and you will be out of luck. So I agreed and then I was elected." Seck's election was unexpected because he is widely viewed as a political outsider and a troublemaker who uses public confrontation as a means of exposing corruption and fraud. A resident of Pikine since 1957, everyone in the neighborhood and in most of Saint Louis knows him as an outspoken critic.

Seck was always eager to be interviewed, and as he pointed out, he wasn't telling me anything that he hadn't said at public meetings or taken to the press, so I should feel free to quote him liberally and use his real name. During our conversations he told story after story about the history of Pikine, and each of his stories turned around the central themes of donor investment, politicization of development projects, and co-option of Pikine's grassroots development efforts by local politicians. "There have been millions of dollars of development initiatives in Pikine," he would begin, "and we have nothing to show for it. Donor funding here has been like water in a leaky bucket. You have to fix the holes if you want to have any water." Most of his criticisms stem from a lack of oversight of major infrastructure projects, and from the failure of project planners and local project managers to account for how donor funding has been spent. In one of his examples the Pikine school received $20,000 to build six new classrooms, but the local school committee could never account for how that money had actually been spent. Seck was convinced that many of these funds had been skimmed from the project budgets, and he was known for making these kinds of accusations at community meetings.

Once Seck became the health committee treasurer he had access to the health post's financial statements and activity reports of the past several years, and he found that there had not been full disclosure of the post's financial situation at the general assembly. His interpretation of the decline of the dispensary stems from the account he pieced together by looking through the books. He laid the majority of the blame on the medical personnel, in particular the head nurse: "They ate all the money, and they ate all the medicines. When we came on board there were zero drugs, zero finances, and lots of bills to be paid." Rather than paying the auxiliary staff (cashier, night guardian) a percentage of the monthly profits (i.e., allowing the market to determine their salaries as mandated by the new management framework), the health committee had also incurred numerous debts to pay them a minimal salary every month. The staff and health committee also regularly reported unusual expenses (US $100 worth of gas when the post had no car or motorbike, or $80 under the category of miscellaneous) that often surpassed the post's monthly earnings. The established precedent seemed to be to spend money first and justify it afterwards. These habits had over the course of several years turned a surplus of US $2,000 to a debt of approximately $1,000.

In spite of a multitude of poor management practices that led to the post's bankruptcy, Seck argued that the main problem was that the medical staff would abuse their access to free medicines, regularly helping themselves to dozens of doses worth of aspirin, chloroquine, and other medicines stocked at the post. The staff would then report this as drug sales, instead of losses, so the pharmaceutical stock would slowly dwindle with no parallel income to replace the drug supply. After months of this happening the health post experienced drug shortages and had no money for resupply.

As treasurer, Seck emphasized that he was first and foremost concerned with combating the practices that led to the post's bankruptcy. He was particularly annoyed that the head nurse and several members of the previous health committee had cellular telephones, which he took as a sure sign of corruption. Seck lobbied the new health committee to use a rigorous accounting approach in which the treasurer and adjunct-treasurer visit the health post daily. They began collecting the post's earnings several times a week and depositing them immediately into the health post bank account. He also lobbied the medical staff to stop raiding the health post pharmacy. In Seck's words: "You can't be sick and go to the dispensary and they give you ten doses of chloroquine, and then the nurse gets sick and takes hundreds. They had to be taking the medicine for themselves and selling it under the table to patients in the consultation rooms." As Turshen points out in her overview of health reform in southern Africa, user fees "actively create commerce" as poorly paid medical staff tap into the new climate of profit making by charging for free services or selling scarce medical supplies for private gain (Turshen 1999, 50). Seck sought to combat this underground privatization of the health post's supplies by making sure that all of the drugs leaving the dispensary's pharmacy were properly accounted for as either sales or free meds for the staff. His hope was that this practice would prevent the staff from taking undue advantage of their right to free medical treatment.

Seck's other major concern was the way that staff would abuse the availability of free care for those with indigent status. He argued that the medical personnel would routinely claim indigent status for friends, relatives, and neighbors who would then receive free care and free drugs at the health post. Together these practices were a steady drain on the health post's profits and eventually caused its demise. In his mind the previous health committees bore little responsibility for the health post's bankruptcy; they had misunderstood the financial management tools but had not intentionally siphoned off medicine or money.

True to his reputation in the neighborhood, Seck used his mastery of the health post's financial record to accuse the medical personnel of theft and corruption. In one exchange, he pointed out that the medical staff were turning in receipt after receipt with no evidence that bills had been paid or goods had been purchased. "Where are the bills? I call that embezzlement, I call that stealing. Abdu says I can't prove that they stole money. I told him, 'You studied law at the university, so sue me.' He says he didn't want it to go that far, so I said, 'Then you really did steal!' I was really trying to provoke him to try to sue me."

While Seck did not square off against the medical personnel in court, he took advantage of several public venues to levy his accusations. He was one of the most vocal critics of the medical personnel at the district orientation for newly elected health committee presidents and treasurers. His ability to recite the exact tally of the health post's expenses and debts caused alarm among some of the district administrators. In their report back to the medical personnel at the following staff meeting, one administrator told the group: "The most dangerous was the Pikine treasurer. He claims people go to the post and there is no one there; that the head nurse doesn't arrive until 11 A.M. He made claims about mismanaging the clinic funds. He had exact figures from his own health post and several others. He had lots of precise information about financial management. I thought he was reading from notes but he had it all in his head." The message to the medical staff was clear: these health committees are watching closely so you must be vigilant and follow the rules. Seck had succeeded at "shaking things up" as he had hoped to do.

This performance at the district meeting caught the attention of the medical district administrators, but Seck continued to be frustrated by the lack of action being taken against Abdu. He reasoned that if Dr. Faal was reviewing each health post's monthly reports, he should have known about Pikine's situation and put an end to the sloppy accounting practices. In his most aggressive move, Seck finally took his allegations to the local radio station, Fréquence-Terenga, which aired his statements and then Abdu's counterallegations of theft by other medical personnel in the district, particularly the hospital personnel. In way of explanation for his approach, Seck commented: "I don't want the dishonest folks to feel safe anymore, we have to shake things up. Because a Senegalese, he only fears two things, the radio and the newspaper." After this explosive confrontation, Dr. Faal mediated a truce and reestablished a working relationship between the Pikine health committee and the head nurse. The medical district agreed to loan the Pikine health post US $1,000 worth of pharmaceuticals, and Seck's rigorous accounting practices and the renewed efforts of the medical staff slowly began to produce results.

"Our health post is sick."—Daba Joob

There were of course competing explanations for how the Pikine dispensary arrived at such a sorry state of affairs. The post's midwife, Daba Joob, argued that nearly all of the post's problems stem from its location.[2] When she first started working, the post was located in a rented house on Angle Taal, one of the two main thoroughfares that runs through the center of Pikine. In 1993 the Partenariat Lille-Saint Louis, one of the most visible donor organizations in the city, agreed to construct a new dispensary for Pikine.[3] After long and heated negotiations about the ideal location for the post, a site in the interior of Pikine was selected. This negotiation was a battle between the two main political parties, the ruling party PS and the opposition PDS, both of which were seeking to offer the dispensary to their constituents as a political favor.

Daba's complaints about the clinic location were related to the impossibility of using public transportation to get there. Taxis were the only option, and most taxi drivers refuse to drive on Pikine's sandy paths. Those who would go there charged seventy cents, as opposed to the flat fare of fifty cents to get anywhere else in Saint Louis. Pikine residents who use public transportation take car-rapides, which follow a set route through the city and cost five cents (US). When confronted with a twenty-minute walk or an expensive cab ride to the Pikine dispensary, most residents choose to walk to the main road and then pay five cents to get to another health post or to the hospital. Women's daily routines take them to the paved road to do their marketing every morning, and most find it more convenient to visit a health post en route rather than returning to the heart of Pikine after they have finished their errands. Daba observed that there has been a drop in utilization rates since the post was moved to Pikine's inaccessible center.

In addition to its remoteness, the health post was constructed near the shallow, central part of Pikine that borders the floodplains of the Senegal River. Seck, always quick to lodge accusations, argued that the annual problems with flooding are a clear indication of the corruption of local officials and the contractors who built the clinic. The feasibility studies and architectural plans should have accounted for flooding and provided adjustments such as raising the building several feet above typical flood levels. As thousands of dollars (US) were spent on the project, he concluded that the absence of such basic flood prevention measures suggests that funds were embezzled or diverted from the building project. As it stands, the Pikine health post is closed two to three months of the year during the rainy season, the very period during which Pikine residents experience the highest rates of malaria, diarrheal disease, and other waterborne illnesses.

Beyond problems with Pikine's geography and topography, the dispensary suffers from the demoralization of its medical staff, which manifests itself in their irregular work habits. The staff often fail to open the clinic on time, and some days the clinic never opens at all. Daba admitted that many of the neighborhood complaints about the health post are true. She described the entire health post as being sick. She described her own attitude toward the post: "Every day when I have to get up and get myself all the way to the health post, I feel discouraged." Numbering among her complaints are the seventy cents (US) she pays in cab fare to and from the health post, and the fact that this money is not reimbursed by the health committee. Daba also complained that the health committee does not give the staff regular bonuses, which might motivate them to work harder. She spoke enviously of hospital employees who work hard, bring in lots of profits, and are rewarded for this work by bonuses from the hospital health committee.[4] Her despair over the state of the Pikine dispensary is understandable, yet she failed to see the connection between the staff's poor habits, mismanagement of clinic funds, the depleted stock of pharmaceuticals, and the low usage rates by Pikine residents.

"There are a lot of politics here."—Abdu Joob

The beleaguered head nurse of the Pikine health post, Abdu Joob, was the subject of much intrigue, discussion, and suspicion in the district, and he was an elusive character during my time in Saint Louis.[5] Many members of the district's fourteen health committees thought that he was directly responsible for the problems in Pikine. They claimed he had "eaten" the post's money and sold the drugs under the table. There was some predictability to these accusations given Pikine's reputation as being one of the most backward and unruly neighborhoods in Saint Louis. Why shouldn't the Pikine health post be plagued with problem after problem, from flooding to bankruptcy to an unmotivated if not wholly corrupt head nurse?

I pursued an interview with Abdu for months with no luck chasing him down. We would greet each other at the district staff meetings and he would feign disappointment that I hadn't come to interview him yet, but somehow we never managed to find a time to meet. I was finally able to interview him after nearly eight months in Saint Louis. At the time of our conversation, the Pikine health post was slowly making its way out of bankruptcy due to the vigilant accounting of the health committee and the redoubled efforts of the medical staff. I suspect that Abdu, who knew of my interviews with the Pikine health committee members and Dr. Faal, avoided being interviewed until the health post's most acute problems were largely resolved. Abdu's own turnaround happened at the staff meeting in April, when Dr. Faal chided him for being provoked by Seck to issue his own allegations of corruption on the local radio. At the end of the meeting, Abdu made a public declaration that he was going to turn his health post around, and he vowed that within a few months the Pikine dispensary was going to be in the top five in the district. His statement was met with the cheers of his fellow head nurses, and he seemed committed to reviving the health post.

During our interview Abdu demonstrated a keen understanding of neighborhood politics, and he acknowledged that the Pikine health post, and the neighborhood in general, ought to be doing much better than they were. "Our job here ought to be easy. You can't come to Pikine and pretend that you know more than the people who live here. The task at hand is really just to coordinate things, because there are some real brains here; all you have to do is come here and do the job you were given to do." Although Pikine residents have the human capital to accomplish development work in the neighborhood, he argued that political divisions and rivalries were the root of Pikine's stagnation. At annual meetings for the health post, senior men and junior men would square off, each accusing the other of holding up progress in the neighborhood. He also mentioned jousting between the two main political parties, and how each sought to capture seats on all of the local boards and committees. In response to my questions about the absence of women on the health committees, he reported that every year they tried to get women on the roster, but in the years that women won positions they rarely finished their terms. Their preference for income-generating activities and their lack of free time made it nearly impossible for them to participate.

Beyond politics, Abdu made a strong case that the Bamako Initiative, with its emphasis on cost recovery through user fees and the sale of generic medicines, was inappropriate for impoverished neighborhoods like Pikine. His conviction confirms the assertion that decentralization fosters inequities. When neighborhoods and medical districts are supposed to cover their own costs in a decentralized health system, there is a strong likelihood that "the districts with the poorest people could provide only the poorest services" (Turshen 1999, 56). Abdu was convinced that Pikine needed donor funding to supplement the meager profits that the health post could make from selling consultation tickets and drugs. In spite of the minimal price of consultation fees, Abdu knew that many Pikine residents saw this as a barrier: "If you have only one dollar in your pocket for the day, you don't want to take twenty-five cents and spend it on a consultation. People need to eat. It is only when they get really sick, then they will be willing to skip eating and go pay for the consultation." As evidence of their small profit margins, Abdu told me that in the four months since the new health committee was elected, they had worked extremely hard and had managed to bring in about US $400 per month. Although this indicated significant progress for Pikine, he felt that Pikine would never be able to meet all of its primary health care needs through the activities of the health post alone.

In Abdu's mind Pikine's location on the outskirts of the city and its large population (unofficial estimates put the population at over 50,000) also require a different strategy from the other urban health posts that were serving 10,000 to 15,000 people. "You can't really consider Pikine an urban dispensary. I have people coming to find me day and night. We don't have a maternity ward and there are too many home births. People have the same transport problems and economic barriers that prevent rural folks from seeking emergency care at the hospital." After living and working in the neighborhood for five years, he was convinced that a rural health post model that provided housing for the head nurse and facilities for assisting women in childbirth was a better model of primary care for Pikine.

I asked Abdu what factors he thought were the most significant in the health post's fall into bankruptcy, and what role he thought the medical personnel had played in this crisis. He responded that the professional staff did play a role, but he put their responsibility at 5 to 10 percent of the total problem, and he again alluded to his assertion that cost recovery can't work in poor neighborhoods. However, though he initially denied much responsibility for the dispensary's problems, he then spoke candidly of his frustration and lack of interest in working in Pikine.[6] He mentioned Pikine's distinction of being the poorest and most populous neighborhood in Saint Louis, and he felt he had received a very undesirable assignment when he was sent to work there. He explains:

> There was a time when I was really unmotivated. In a professional sense, I really wanted to apply myself but sometimes you look at the advantages of your colleagues compared to yourself, when you have such a large population. You are really discouraged. You say you don't have a damn thing to do here and you are going to go work somewhere else.[7] But at the end of the day, if you do this you are only hurting yourself, because you turn your post into a bad post. This is what happened to me. But now, I am in the process of showing them that I can do better, because I have the physical, intellectual, and moral capacity. I am no longer going to succumb to discouragement. Right now I am motivated, I am showing what I am capable of.

Abdu was filled with a sense of injustice at having been assigned to Pikine while his colleagues, who often made Pikine the butt of their jokes, had more enviable positions in better neighborhoods.

Living and working in Pikine seemed to threaten Abdu's pride in his professional training. At the close of our interview he emphasized that he comes from a medical family and that he had received the best nursing training from distinguished professors. It is this sense of pride, shared widely among medical professionals, that often contributes to their reticence in working with the health committees. Not only are these committee members seen as being from a lower, less-educated social class, they are often overzealous in their duties and tend to regard themselves as the supervisors of the medical personnel. Effective collaboration between medical professionals and community members is difficult to mandate from above, particularly when medical staff already feel besieged by their dire working conditions and miserable salaries.

Nonetheless, Abdu was coaxed by the Pikine health committee to redeem himself, the health post, and Pikine by returning to work and maintaining a positive attitude. After much negotiation and mediation by Dr. Faal, the Pikine health post began its slow recovery. By the end of 1999 the post's earnings were close to US $400 per month, although the monthly overhead was often very close to this amount. Although some of the district posts have thousands of dollars in surplus profits, many months the Pikine post is barely able to recover its costs.

Pikine as a Reflection of Tensions in the Medical District

The Pikine health post, with its slow descent into bankruptcy and increasing antagonism between the medical staff and health committee, offers a glimpse into the weaknesses of the decentralized health system. There was widespread consensus in the neighborhood that the quality of care at the health post was poor, that it was often closed, and that its remote location and user fees constituted real barriers to seeking services there. The medical staff's own low regard for the health post was evident in Abdu and Daba's visible frustration with having been assigned to work in Pikine. Neither of them acknowledged abusing their access to free pharmaceuticals, but it is not difficult to imagine how the low morale and abysmal pay of medical staff can spiral into mismanagement of health resources. The contentious relations between the health committee and the health post staff reveal one of the main vulnerabilities of the new system of community management. Instead of achieving a collaborative partnership, a dysfunctional health committee and a frustrated staff oversaw the collapse of the health post. Pikine is a unique case given the severity of its problems; several other city health posts flirted occasionally with debt, but no case was as dire or as chronic as Pikine's.

In spite of these particularities, the factors that contributed to the dispensary's bankruptcy are not uncommon in the district or the health system. Health committees are not elected democratically, and they often have political motives. This finding is not unique to Senegal. Other studies have found that "decentralization leads to strengthening of prevailing political domination, whether by controlling political conflict, reinforcing local patronage systems, or extending central control over local government" (Turshen 1999, 56; Collins and Green 1994). Many in Saint Louis viewed the seats on the health committees as an opportunity for political parties and aspiring politicians to gain access to medical supplies and cash and to offer access to medical care in exchange for party loyalty. The location of the health post itself had been determined by competition between the two main political parties, each of which wanted to claim that it had secured the new health post (a donor-funded project) for its constituency.

Beyond the politicization of the health committees, throughout the Saint Louis medical district there was ongoing tension between health committees and medical personnel. The state of flux and transition in the health care system and the lack of understanding of some of the significant reforms facilitated many of these conflicts. "Loose" financial management on the part of the head nurses and the committees was widespread, and the mutual lack of trust between medical personnel and committee members fostered frequent confrontations. The main distinction between Pikine and other health structures was that in most health posts these conflicts would flare up and then be extinguished, while in Pikine the situation smoldered for months until the final blaze resulted in total bankruptcy.

Pikine's experience reflects the multiple factors that determine the success of a medical structure. In theory, the system of health committees mark a step toward community participation in the health system, and it represents an effort to allow health needs to be defined by local settings, a highly desirable outcome of reform (Janes 2004). The recent reforms and transformations have created confusion about the authority and financial responsibilities of the district supervisor, municipal authorities, and community partners. Within this realm negotiations and overt conflict occur between the district administrators, their staff, and the health committees. This transition period created an arena within which various players in the health sector do battle for status, power, and the social and material advantages of involvement in the health posts. While rules and regulations provide a theoretical mode of operation, many actors take it upon themselves to maneuver and negotiate the rules to their advantage. Pikine's experience confirms assertions that the mere inclusion of "community" or "civil society" in the health system is no guarantee of equitable outcomes, as these categories "can obscure varieties of social inequality: class, ethnicity, and gender" (Janes 2004, 463). As the primary consumer of health care services, women have been notably absent from the new community management structures (Foley 2001). In Pikine a history of mistrust, evidence of mismanagement, and lack of accountability on the part of professional staff and committee members crippled meaningful citizen participation in the health post.

The eventual recovery of the Pikine health post illustrates that even in the face of numerous constraints, medical personnel and health committees can have a tremendous impact on the success or failure of medical structures. If head nurses and health committees collaborate effectively and apply the guidelines of the Bamako Initiative, even dispensaries in very poor neighborhoods can usually recover enough of their costs to ensure their ongoing operation. Although there is evidence that cost recovery is neither efficient nor effective at financing health systems (Creese 1990; Turshen 1999), health posts that don't recover their costs risk being shut down or languishing in bankruptcy until a donor or the medical district can bail them out. The partnership between the head nurses and the health committees is the crux of the health care system's success, and this relationship has proven difficult. Overzealous or incompetent committees frequently alienate the head nurses, who often view the health committees with a certain degree of resentment and reticence. When these potential pitfalls are overcome, the dispensaries tend to run smoothly. Yet the poor reputations of many neighborhood health posts, and the social distance between medical personnel and patients, create additional barriers to using the city's health posts. These and other obstacles to seeking care are the focus of chapters 7 and 8.

6

Knowledge Encounters

Biomedicine, Islam, and Wolof Medicine

Health sector reform in Senegal created new social spaces for the management and delivery of biomedical care, as well as new kinds of relationships between medical professionals and community members. To date there have been tremendous discrepancies between the envisioned benefits of decentralization and community management of health facilities and the contentious arena within which different social actors maneuver to control resources and accrue social capital. A similar disjuncture exists between the expectations of biomedical professionals and the actual health strategies of Saint Louis and Ganjool residents.

The most obvious collision between health-seeking practices and the assumptions of biomedical providers is conveyed by the notion of *responsibilization*, which implies the expectation that people should be responsible for themselves. These appeals to "empowering" citizens to take responsibility for their health came to prominence with the implementation of the Bamako Initiative, which itself was the result of pressure on African governments to find new solutions to health care shortages in light of declining budgets. The responsibilization discourse has been fully incorporated into state and NGO rhetoric about overcoming Senegal's health challenges. Implicit in this idea of "becoming responsible" is the liberal assumption that individuals are rational and conscious decision makers whose health actions are unfettered by social or cultural constraints. This image of the freely acting "neoliberal subject" has been inherent to the logic of market-based health reforms (Blas and Hearst 2001; Foley 2008). In contrast, people in Saint Louis are bound up in complex webs of relations and they occupy social locations that have a direct influence on their knowledge of illness and their therapeutic options.

While health programs typically assume that most of the population, and women in particular, must be convinced to engage in preventative and curative

96

health behavior, men and women from all socioeconomic backgrounds spend an extraordinary amount of time, energy, and money pursuing good health. As in much of sub-Saharan Africa, biomedicine in Senegal coexists alongside many other modes of medical knowledge often characterized as "indigenous," "local," or "traditional" (Feierman and Janzen 1992; Janzen 1978; Lambek 1993; Luedke and West 2006; Vaughan 1991). Islam and Christianity offer additional frameworks for addressing issues of sickness and health. Accordingly, a large portion of health-seeking behavior in Senegal, both curative and preventative, takes place outside of biomedical frameworks (Fassin 1992; Fassin and Fassin 1988; Keita 1996). These health strategies often remain invisible to biomedical observers, many of whom argue that the solution to Senegal's health dilemmas lies in greater acceptance and use of biomedicine. This chapter challenges these hegemonic understandings of Senegal's illness landscape and demonstrates how people's health practices stem from encounters between biomedicine, Islam, and Wolof medicine. Chapters 7 and 8 explore the ways that stratified social relations shape people's ability to make use of these different therapeutic frameworks.

Conceptualizing Medical Pluralism and Senegalese Healing Traditions

In the summer of 1999 the administrative and clinical personnel of the Saint Louis medical district were in the midst of an ongoing epidemic. In recent years there had been an overabundance of middle-aged women seeking treatment for hypertension, which Wolof speakers in Saint Louis refer to as *tension*. Almost every day I would hear women describing a whole host of medical problems that could be explained by their tension going up or down. Some women took their tension more seriously than others and made the rounds of the city's health posts, military clinic, and hospital seeking relief from their symptoms. Hypertension, when diagnosed by a biomedical provider, is known to require regular monitoring of one's blood pressure. At each clinical encounter women would insist that the nurses strap the blood pressure sleeve around their arms and give them their reading. If this was not done, women insisted that they had not been examined thoroughly. As one women exclaimed: "How can they say they have given you a medical exam, when they've got instruments right there that they aren't even using on you!" These complaints about their medical consultations for tension reflect more general observations about the city's health posts. Women object to the perceived low quality of services and the stubborn medical personnel who do not meet their expectations about clinical encounters.

The rising popularity of hypertension as a biomedical diagnosis and women's interest in monitoring their blood pressure reflect the interplay between emerging chronic diseases and traditional Wolof standards of beauty.

Hypertension, in all likelihood due to its association with obesity, has become a new social marker for women in Saint Louis. In traditional standards of feminine beauty, Wolof women of a certain age should aspire to be well groomed, slow moving, laden in gold, and draped in expensive fabrics sewn in traditional female styles. Above all they should be large, or even very large.[1] These women, known as *drianke*, have near mythic reputations as seductive, powerful, and potentially dangerous women (Nyamnjoh 2005). In alluding to their tension going up and down, women in Saint Louis assert their likeness to these cultural symbols of female beauty and power. Part of enacting this cultural and medical claim involves the conspicuous consumption of biomedical services and the ritual of having one's blood pressure taken.

For their part, the medical personnel in Saint Louis were exasperated with the popular claim to be hypertensive because they were having problems keeping blood pressure sleeves in stock—many of the women seeking blood pressure readings were so large that the standard sleeves could not fit around their arms. The nurses and nurses' aides, in an attempt to comply with the high demand for blood pressure checks, kept breaking their instruments. This was not the kind of self-advocacy and "taking responsibility for one's health" that health planners imagined when they called for greater patient participation in managing health problems. The tension epidemic illuminates how biomedical knowledge and technologies are filtered through existing understandings of the body and illness. Tension is neither a wholly biomedical nor "local" disease, but the product of interactions between a biomedical disease construction and Wolof understandings of health, beauty, and womanhood.

Historical and contemporary encounters between biomedicine, Islam, and local healing traditions have produced the cultural repertoires that rural and urban women use to promote health. Biomedicine stands as one option among many, including Wolof medicine, a broad category including Islamic practitioners as well as herbalists, diviners, mocckat, and others (Fassin 1992; Keita 1996). Many studies of medical pluralism in sub-Saharan Africa attempt to classify practitioners, remedies, and preventative and curative strategies into the broad categories of biomedicine and traditional medicine, or to distinguish between formal health institutions (public and private) and informal structures (Beckerleg 1994; Janzen 1978; Keita 1996). This tradition has a long history in Africanist scholarship that sought to describe "African systems of thought" as distinct from Western science and rationality (Evans-Pritchard 1937; Horton 1967).

To some extent these analytic divisions match the ways that people themselves describe local medical options; Senegalese can easily identify illnesses that should be treated by biomedicine (*garab u tubaab*) versus those that require Wolof medicine (*garab u Wolof*). Leach et al.'s (2008) recent research in Guinea transcends these standard categories of classification by addressing how patients themselves, in this case parents seeking care for sick children, evaluate different medical options. They argue that common analytic distinctions between traditional and modern, and public and private medicine "occlude the identification of the distinctions that are actually relevant to people as they seek health" (Leach et al. 2008, 2158). Although people can readily make use of the traditional versus modern binary, this categorization may have little significance when making treatment decisions. Within the Guinean therapeutic landscape the most salient distinctions include the following: providers who treat men's illnesses versus those of women and children; ailments with known remedies versus those that require expert diagnosis; illnesses treatable by injection; the types of payment accepted; the quality of the medicine; and whether medicine is strong or weak (Leach et al. 2008, 2159). Some of these criteria are equally relevant in the Senegalese context, particularly the difference between familiar and unknown illnesses, and the type of payment and the timing of payment for services.

In his classic review essay on studies of African healing systems, Feierman (1985) argues that historically there have been three conceptual approaches to African therapeutic traditions; each approach addresses how therapeutic choices are made and who controls the therapeutic process. In one approach the emphasis is on shared values, "each society, the argument goes, has its own body of cultural knowledge for the interpretation of illness" (Feierman 1985, 76). Within this perspective there are different understandings of the extent to which knowledge traditions are "open" or "closed," and the degree to which patients and healers respect boundaries between different medical systems. Anthropological studies of medical pluralism often treated medical traditions as closed systems, yet therapeutic traditions that "travel" are transformed as they become incorporated into particular medical landscapes. In her historical work on medicine in southern Africa, Vaughan argues that biomedicine is just as "African" as any other African therapeutic tradition (1991). Fassin's (1992) ethnography of healing and health seeking in a Dakar suburb emphasizes the ways that biomedicine has been "indigenized" in Senegal, while Keita's (2006) work emphasizes the extent to which all of the religious and ethnomedical traditions in Senegal have influenced one another over the past several centuries.

In addition to recognizing the interactions of various medical systems, Feierman stresses the importance of "the coexistence of multiple explanations in each African society and in each individual's thought" (1985, 76). Last (1992) suggests that the boundaries between medical traditions are often of little significance to lay people, since patients in northern Nigeria use multiple therapies with very little concern for "coherent medical tradition." Fassin (1992) adds that medical anthropologists often overestimate the importance of boundaries and attribute an unwarranted degree of systematicity and coherence to healing traditions. His research suggests that the logic of therapeutic itineraries is often only decipherable in hindsight, and that many Senegalese patients take a pragmatic approach and make use of multiple therapies (Fassin 1992). Saint Louis residents refer to this approach as *lambatu*, that is, trying anything that one thinks might work with little concern for the type of expertise that might bring relief from illness.

Leach et al.'s (2008) research in Guinea supports Last's contention that the perceived efficacy of a particular therapy and its appropriateness for the ailment in question can overshadow distinctions between different medical systems. There is much ethnographic evidence that practitioners and patients frequently consult across lines of ethnicity, language, and social class, which calls into question the notion of bounded knowledge or "closed" systems. Moving beyond the "bounded systems" approach to medical pluralism (Brodwin 1996; Janzen 1978; Obbo 1996), research in southern Africa emphasizes the social processes that allow for the active maintenance and crossing of therapeutic borders (Luedke and West 2006). Most contemporary scholarship is in agreement that boundaries between medical traditions are fluid at best, and that both patients and practitioners frequently exercise their ability to move between and among different healing frameworks.

A second set of approaches to African medical systems emphasizes competition among healers (Feierman 1985). This competition revolves around who has the power to legitimate disease and to excuse the patient from work and other social responsibilities. In the contentious field of diagnosing and interpreting illness, healers assert the supremacy of their skill and healing expertise vis-à-vis their competitors. Fassin's (1992) work applies Foucauldian notions of power-knowledge to explore how Senegalese healers deploy different kinds of therapeutic power. The more powerful the healer, the more likely that therapy will have an oral dimension, such as spoken prayer, benedictions, and the like. In contrast, less powerful healers make greater use of amulets and medicinal plants (Fassin 1992). Senegalese often rely on word of mouth to assess the potency of particular therapies, and this kind of information tends to be much more important in therapeutic decisions than healers' assertions about their skills. This finding echoes Feierman's argument that analysis of competition among healers fails to recognize that patient and family make important decisions about the nature of the illness before consulting with a practitioner (1985, 79).

Feierman's third approach to studying African health and healing examines how a patient's relatives and neighbors control the therapeutic process by choosing among many therapeutic options. Building on Janzen's (1978) ethnography of the "quest for therapy" in the former Zaire he emphasizes that while healers may offer a variety of choices for therapy, therapy-managing groups ultimately determine the course of action. Therefore "the people who make the most crucial therapeutic decisions tend not to have expert medical knowledge, whether in the biomedical or popular medical sphere" (Feierman 1985, 82). This recognition reiterates the importance of understanding how lay people understand health and illness, as their perceptions of risk, vulnerability, and efficacy are crucial in determining treatment options. Perhaps most relevant to the politics of medical decision making in Senegal, "the authority of lay therapy managers is not separate from generalized authority in the domestic and community sphere, all the factors which shape local communities affect healing" (Feierman 1985, 82). Such a statement reminds us to place issues of health and healing within socioeconomic contexts in order to analyze the interplay of social hierarchies and medical care. In chapters 7 and 8 we will see the gendered and generational politics of therapy management, as male heads of households allocate therapeutic resources as they see fit, while women have little ability to shape medical itineraries.

Senegal's history of Islamization, French conquest and colonization, and the presence of many ethnomedical traditions have produced a therapeutically rich and diverse setting in which to pursue good health. While one can identify different medical traditions—biomedicine, Islam, Wolof medicine—there are fluid boundaries between these frameworks that are crossed frequently by healers and patients alike. Originally a French import, biomedicine has been localized throughout the twentieth century, and there are public, private, formal, and informal biomedical practitioners. French civil servants once dominated many of the prestigious medical posts in government and in the elite medical structures, but Senegalese physicians have moved to prominent positions within the medical school, teaching hospitals, and the Ministry of Health. A wide gap remains between the biomedical knowledge of experts and that of the lay public, but vaccines, shots, and pharmaceuticals are familiar and popular medical treatments that have become part of daily routines of health seeking.

Given the early arrival of Islam in Senegal, and the resilience of Muslim Sufi orders throughout the colonial period and to the present day, it is unsurprising that Islam offers Senegalese a rich repertoire for therapeutic action. In contemporary Senegal the Sufi *tariqa* are an important feature of religious and social life, and regular participation in pilgrimages, rites, and rituals of these orders is a cornerstone of health practice. Islam of course has a long history and a written corpus of legal, scientific, and medical texts, and it must be recognized as an independent tradition, yet in Senegal it has saturated all aspects of social life. There were medical and therapeutic traditions in Senegal prior to widespread acceptance of Islam, and a few specific therapies such as *ndëp* (exorcism of traditional spirits) seem to be relatively free from Islamic influence. However, the bulk of what most people would call traditional medicine, aggregated under the broad category "Wolof medicine," is suffused with Islamic knowledge and practice.

Within each therapeutic framework are many sources of information and modes of knowledge circulation; as people seek solutions to health problems they often solicit the expertise of doctors, nurses, lay midwives, diviners, or *sëriñ* (Muslim marabouts). Information and knowledge about particular therapists and therapies circulate in the form of stories and anecdotes. Certain illnesses, such as malaria, receive little attention, while stories of witchcraft, possession, and evil spirits abound and are a primary concern for rural and urban folks alike. Vehicles of popular culture such as radio, television, and print media are arenas in which people debate what it means to be "well" in the broadest sense, from being a good spouse to a good parent and a devout Muslim. Rural and urban dwellers are regularly exposed to health messages coming from the Ministry of Health, NGOs, and other development agencies. Each of these actors uses education campaigns to promote certain understandings of diseases such as malaria and HIV/AIDS, and to encourage the population to take certain kinds of preventative and curative health actions.

In light of these multiple frameworks for understanding disease, there are varied patterns of health seeking. While people have different understandings of Islamic laws and religious practice, all Senegalese Muslims would agree that they are trying to fulfill Islamic ideals. People in town are more exposed to biomedical health messages than their rural counterparts, largely through the medium of television, billboards, and print media, and biomedical concepts of disease are more apparent in daily conversations about health in Saint Louis. But whereas biomedicine lends itself to the quick resolution of certain illnesses such as malaria, it contributes very little to preventative health strategies in town or in the village where a range of approaches may be used.

Therapeutic Landscapes and Health Practice in the Saint Louis Region

While the local reformulation of some biomedical illness categories such as tension have taken on a life of their own, Senegalese medical professionals constantly lament the lack of seriousness with which many people regard other endemic diseases. The most problematic disease is malaria, which kills more adults and children every year than any other ailment. Throughout the summer of 1999 the entire Ganjool region was gripped by an unusually severe malaria outbreak. Generous rains submerged the road to Saint Louis under several meters of water and made it impassable for about eight weeks. Malaria deaths spiked, and the flooding and unusable road served as a constant reminder of Ganjool's marginal status. The heavy rains coincided with my attempts to conduct a household demographic census in Mumbaay. As I walked from house to house asking about family members, births, deaths, and ages of children, I began to wonder how many members of each household I would find lying motionless in the courtyard on straw mats. Sometimes it was a few children, sometimes a parent and several children, and in the worst cases I would find several adults and children all lying completely immobile, hoping to sweat out the sickness. For eight weeks the village was literally knocked flat on its back with malarial fever.

Throughout the rainy season I was not the only one whose heart would stop when verses from the Koran sounded out over the mosque loudspeaker, followed by the gravelly voice of a village elder who would call out the name of the latest victim of *sibiiru* (malaria). In a span of four weeks the village of 1,200 lost ten people. With every death all activities would come to a halt and men would gather to bury the dead while women paid their condolences to the deceased's household. As one of the teenage boys in my household commented, it seemed to the men that as soon as they returned from burying the latest victim the loudspeaker would call out again. In spite of the high death toll there was no general sense of alarm or panic in the village—sibiiru was an old foe that had lost its ability to elicit much reaction of any kind from young or old. Most people did not use bed nets, and they did not take chloroquine at the first sign of fever during the rainy season. The Wolof word for malaria, sibiiru, has become a general gloss to describe all kinds of ailments from mild headaches and fever to full-blown malaria requiring immediate biomedical attention. The village health workers lamented that *danu xeb sibiiru*, people just don't fear malaria. Most people would get sibiiru many times in their life, and most would survive.

The malaria outbreak was one of many occasions that sparked the frustration of the village health hut workers. The health hut is the only medical facility in Daru-Mumbaay, and it opened in 1984 as part of the medical district's attempt to extend primary health care to the rural areas surrounding Saint Louis. The village elders selected Sali Jah and Khadi Geye to serve as the village birth assistants and community health workers. They began work in the village after a training period of twelve months at Ganjool's only health dispensary in Tassinère. Since the end of their training, Sali and Khadi have been assisting births, providing first aid, selling essential medicines (chloroquine, aspirin, oral rehydration packets), and complaining about the often lackadaisical attitude of their fellow villagers toward malaria, infant malnutrition, and other common village maladies.

On many days I would walk with Khadi Geye to the health hut located in the center of the village. Often there were few patients, and as she explained: "Some days you are just sitting in the breeze. You just sit here all day and you don't make a dime." It was always interesting to watch the day's medical consultations, but there were long empty hours to whittle away with conversations about village health problems. Working on a near-volunteer basis as community health agents was nothing if not aggravating for both Sali and Khadi. They are supposed to receive a small percentage of the health hut's monthly profit, but given the minuscule cash flow into the health hut they essentially work for free.

Equally frustrating was their observation that most villagers had neither the time nor the cash resources to respond effectively to illness. Their basic biomedical training had taught them that prevention, as well as early action in the face of illness, were essential in treating the most common village ailments. Again and again villagers with sick family members would not respond soon enough, instead waiting until *dafa leen epp doole*, or until the illness had more strength than they did. In Sali's words: "There are women, when their kids are sick, they just sit. They don't bring them in. They don't ask us anything. They just keep working until the illness gets out of hand." Once an illness is out of hand, the usual solution is to evacuate the patient to the dispensary in Tassinère or to the hospital in Saint Louis. While the villagers were often hoping to wait out an illness, Sali and Khadi saw this strategy as an ill-informed delay that would only incur additional time and expense later on.

The health workers frequently complained about lack of early health action, but patients and their families were often pursuing multiple therapeutic routes, only some of which involved biomedical interventions. "Lambatu" (going back and forth) was the word that women used to describe their health actions. This strategy means combining many different kinds of Wolof medicine with biomedicine. This course of pursuing medical treatment was typically described as "doing anything" one could until the illness was resolved or until one simply had to "wait for God." While medical anthropologists have long sought to unravel patients' therapeutic itineraries by documenting serial and simultaneous use of different therapies in the quest for health, women have a very pragmatic understanding of their health strategies. A person will try anything they think might work: "You just lambatu, you get what you can from *tubaab* (Western) medicine and from Wolof medicine. Whatever people tell you works, you will go and try it."

While many people are willing to try any therapy they think might work, others are skeptical of the efficacy of biomedicine and only very reluctantly seek biomedical care. Some Pikine residents reason that because biomedical interventions and biomedical illnesses are relatively new, they lack credibility. They cite the lack of biomedical care in the past as evidence that perhaps these interventions are unnecessary or ineffective. As one focus group participant suggested, "They say the old folks never went to the hospital, they never used to go anywhere, and the kinds of problems that we have today, they didn't have them." Patients sort through conflicting evidence on the efficacy of biomedicine and other therapies as they cope with specific illness episodes. Some women do very little in the way of prenatal or postnatal care and have no problems with pregnancies and delivery, while others are rigorous in attending their prenatal visits, deliver at the hospital, and still have serious problems. This leads many women to conclude "everyone has what they believe in, [and] that's what they do."

Sali and Khadi often found themselves trying to instill a biomedically oriented logic that ran counter to villagers' medical frameworks and collective common sense. For example, in addition to their disregard for malaria, Khadi complained about women's lack of understanding of how to combat malnutrition. She commented: "There are a lot of children that are *xiiboon* [skinny]; there is a lot of malnutrition. It has to do with the diet. It is the mothers who don't pay a lot of attention to what their children are eating. And the things to eat are grown right here! We have carrots, we have beans, we have cabbage, we have fish. All those things are here. The mothers don't give their kids those things to eat. . . . Some of them, if you tell them, they will start paying attention. There are some, even if you tell them, they won't do it." Khadi and Sali frequently described ways of combating infant and child illness that did not correspond with women's ideas about caring for children. This slippage created immense frustration when their medical advice was disregarded or ignored.

In their attempts to combat infant mortality, the village health workers have tried to emphasize the importance of breastfeeding immediately after birth and then exclusively until foods are introduced at six months. One young mother with a newborn scoffed at Sali's instructions that the baby should only be given breast milk for several months. This advice was designed to ensure that the baby received adequate nutrition and did not become sick from dirty water or waterborne illnesses. On the day of her baby's baptism the new mother commented: "Sali said not to give the baby water, but everyone knows that you give babies water." When what "everyone knows" conflicts with the health workers' instructions, chances are that biomedically based knowledge will be discounted. Certain biomedical interventions are commonly accepted, such as using oral rehydration therapy for infant and child diarrhea, and taking iron during pregnancy to combat anemia, but the village health workers have been unable to instill a general predilection for biomedical prevention and treatment among most villagers.

In spite of their annoyance with villagers' treatment decisions, Sali and Khadi recognize the centrality of economic calculations in villagers' health-seeking decisions, particularly as the onion economy continues to decline. When talking about the general lack of enthusiasm about using the health hut, Khadi emphasized that everyone is *baadoolo* (poor), and the poor can't pay for health care. In Sali's words: "There is no way to get care without paying in Senegal. Your pocket is what cures you. If you have nothing in your pocket, you will die." Since most women and men in Mumbaay survive on credit until the onion harvest, they are reluctant to add to their debt for anything but essential items. Women often have little access to cash because their earnings from one harvest never tide them over until the next one.

For the health workers, this recognition of village poverty does not always alleviate their exasperation with people's health actions. Khadi Geye often complained of people who are "cheap" and don't want to pay for the consultation ticket in addition to the medicine. She jokingly described this reticence about paying the health hut fees as "feeling sorry for one's pocket" and therefore waiting as long as possible before spending money on medical treatment. She was also frustrated about poor attendance at the health education sessions held at the health hut: "You call them for meetings and you give them information and some of them believe it and some of them don't." The lack of concern about malaria was a particular grievance of the health workers, as taking nivaquine at the first signs of illness can usually resolve it with no further medical intervention. Although both Sali and Khadi were deeply familiar with the various constraints villagers faced regarding health strategies, their limited biomedical training had instilled in them a conviction about individual responsibility for health and well-being. They found much evidence in the village that men and women were not taking adequate action to respond to health problems.

In contrast to the health workers' sense that their patients were often negligent in the early stages of illness, villagers in Ganjool and shantytown residents in Pikine continually called attention to user fees as a major obstacle to seeking care. The institutionalization of user fees is the most visible change in the mind of would-be patients who now have to pay upfront for medical consultations and pharmaceuticals that were free in the past. In the wake of the privatization of government health services, many people emphasized that without money one cannot get health care. Women see themselves as baadoolo, and they argue that baadoolo have been shut out of the new health care system.

These claims may be true for both rural and urban women, but village women in Mumbaay have fewer options for supplementing their meager resources than women in town who can find work in the informal sector. Although Pikine is economically marginal within Saint Louis, women living there demonstrate a tremendous ability to "make do" and eke out a living with microbusinesses. With a very small investment of capital (often less than US $10) women can buy produce or other goods at wholesale prices and resell them in their immediate neighborhoods. These women meet many of their personal and household needs with very small sums of money, and they have more access to cash than residents of Mumbaay. Women in town also have access to microcredit through organized women's groups and informal rotating savings and credit associations. When it is their turn to receive the group's savings they are able to start a new kind of income-generating activity, take care of existing debts, or resolve other problems.

Nonetheless, in focus group conversations the cost of treatment was a significant concern for town residents in spite of their greater access to the cash economy. Selling clothes and begging in and around the hospital were two strategies that women used to get cash for treatment. Going to a sëriñ instead of a biomedical caregiver is also a way of avoiding the need for cash, as many healers are willing to be paid in-kind, or after the successful resolution of the patient's medical problem. As one woman explained: "You have to use the sëriñ if you have no money. If they [biomedical clinic] give you a prescription that costs US $20, versus if you could go to the healer and get well without paying that much, you are going to do that." Daily life involves numerous calculations in which needs are balanced against periodic costs such as health care or accoutrements for weddings and baptisms. Medical interventions that cost US 20 cents or less, such as mocc or purchasing herbal remedies, can usually be sought with little difficulty. Visits to a clinic, which can include transportation costs, the consultation ticket, and filling prescriptions, require a serious effort to acquire significant sums of money. When husbands are unwilling or unable to furnish these health care costs, women rely on their own credit networks that can include siblings, parents, in-laws, extended kin, and friends.

While urban and rural poverty are significant obstacles to obtaining health care, the cost of treatment represents only one prohibitive aspect of seeking biomedical care. Villagers have distinct preferences between the two health workers, and some revealed a lack of confidence in their know-how and bedside manner. In Mumbaay, nearly everyone prefers to be treated by Khadi Geye, which is unfortunate as her husband lives two hours away in Thiès and she makes regular trips to visit him. During Khadi's absences many people prefer to sit out an illness rather than deal with Sali. As one friend remarked about Sali, "*Xamul jigeen dara*," meaning that she doesn't know anything about women and she has no idea how to treat people respectfully.

Some villagers have a low regard for Khadi's and Sali's medical expertise, and they often dismiss the primary health interventions available at the health hut. They reason that there are no real medicines there and that the health workers have only minimal training. If you are truly sick, the villagers argued, why not go directly to the real nurse in Tassinère or all the way to the hospital in Saint Louis? The relatively close proximity of more sophisticated medical structures worked to minimize perceptions of the health hut's utility. This bias against the health hut becomes a self-fulfilling prophecy, as patients delay treatment until they surpass the level of care available to them from Sali and Khadi. Nonetheless, Sali and Khadi argue that in the twenty years of the health hut's existence they have witnessed significant declines in infant mortality, rates of anemia, and diarrheal diseases as well as increased use of contraceptives and longer birth intervals.

Urban dwellers had similar critiques of the care they received from nurses in the neighborhood health posts in Saint Louis. Women reported dissatisfaction with their clinic visits because of the failure of doctors and nurses to give them a clear diagnosis or to explain prescriptions. In many instances women's expectations about what should happen during the course of a curative consultation at the dispensary or hospital were not met. As one Pikine resident complained: "You can go to the dispensary and they don't have any medicine. And when you go, they don't heal you, they don't examine you." Many women expressed frustration with the tendency of nurses to take the patient's history instead of conducting physical examinations. In the words of another Pikine patient, "Looking and doing an examination are not the same thing. They have to really look at you. They have tools they should put on your body to examine you. They should take all your vital signs. But you go and tell them what is wrong and they glance at you and write you a prescription. When I go they have to examine me, give me a good checkup, look at my body. They should put their instruments on your body, see what is wrong with you, and then write you a prescription." While medical personnel are trained to streamline care by eliciting the patient's major complaint and making a diagnosis, from the perspective of the patients this process fails to determine the real cause of their illness. Pikine residents also complained about the bedside manner of the dispensary nurses and the attending doctors and midwives at the hospital.

In spite of their objections, the close proximity of Saint Louis neighborhoods, each with its own health post, affords town residents some ability to "comparison shop" among clinics and providers. If one is dissatisfied with the quality of care at a particular dispensary it is easy enough to seek treatment at another. Particular doctors, nurses, and midwives have a reputation for being *laabiir* (compassionate), while others are thought to be rude and disrespectful. Women are savvy patients with high expectations about the quality of service they should receive, and they will frequent the dispensaries they believe offer the best care. Though Pikine residents discriminate between the quality of care given at different health structures and by different medical personnel, many of them cannot afford what they perceive to be the highest quality care offered in private clinics or at the hospital. In spite of knowing that better treatment exists elsewhere, they resign themselves to unsatisfactory care and rude treatment by health post nurses, delay treatment, or they seek alternatives to biomedicine.

For residents of Mumbaay, little comparison shopping exists because the obstacles posed by transportation and cost make biomedical care much less accessible. Instead there is a more straightforward calculation in deciding whether to seek biomedical care. For anything more serious than cuts and scrapes or the early signs of malaria, a trip to the Tassinère health post is required. Before heading to the Tassinère dispensary, villagers will try to cope with an illness using local remedies, as such a trip requires an investment of time and money that many villagers simply don't have. After waiting out an illness for several days or even longer, many patients need to be evacuated directly to the hospital in Saint Louis, an even greater ordeal. Some patients and their families never pursue a course of treatment outside of Mumbaay, instead making due with the plethora of local therapies, or turning their fate over to God.

God Is the Medicine for Everything

If the formal health system in Senegal has only been moderately successful in distilling certain kinds of biomedical logic into frameworks for responding to illness, the undoubtedly hegemonic frame of reference is Islam. Islam shapes people's sense of themselves, and their understandings and experiences of illness and healing, in such profound ways that it is nearly impossible to disentangle Islam from the local healing traditions of Senegal's ethnic groups. Daily life in both Saint Louis and Mumbaay is punctuated by performing ablutions and the five prayers. Giving and receiving blessings (from elders, parents, and friends for one's health, wealth, and success in business and marriage) is a crucial part of social discourse and interaction. During the everyday routines of home, work, and leisure, God is invoked constantly in the course of social greetings, exchanging news, talk of the future, and coping with life's challenges.

Women in town and in the village continuously reiterated the importance of faith in daily life: "People have to put themselves in God's hands. Because God says, 'Pray to me and I will give to you.' Even non-Muslims like Catholics, they pray to God . . . whoever God helps will succeed." Within this hegemonic framework there are ongoing debates about *halal* (acceptable) versus *haram* (forbidden) practices, from family planning to using skin bleaching cream to having multiple wives. The resounding consensus is that people must conduct their private and public affairs according to Islamic precepts, but debate and multiple interpretations about the acceptability of certain practices and behaviors are common.

If there were once distinct medical traditions such as divination, herbalism, and therapies to treat mental illness and spirit possession, to name a few, the centuries-long process of Islamization in Senegal has meant that many local therapies now incorporate religious dimensions (Fassin 1992; Keita 2006). Few lay people distinguish between the healing powers of Islamic experts and the infusion of Muslim prayers and mystical knowledge into other kinds of healing techniques. The Wolof word for imam or Muslim cleric (*sëriñ*) has largely replaced the Wolof word for healer (*fajjkat*); when pursuing nonbiomedical treatment, people often say that they are going to the sëriñ to get Wolof medicine. Special prayers are often part of the process of gathering, preparing, and administering herbal remedies. Prayer and seeking the blessings of religious experts are common health strategies. Annual pilgrimages to the holy sites of Senegal's Sufi orders, and fulfilling religious duties of alms giving and charity, are means of protecting oneself and enhancing one's spiritual, physical, and material well-being.

Most Senegalese seek Islamic protection from spirits, supernatural beings, and other malevolent forces (Fassin 1992). In contemporary Senegal, Islamic ideas about evil spirits such as *jinne* overlap with non-Islamic entities like *rabb* (ancestral spirits) and *dëm* (shape-shifters that consume human flesh). In Wolof tradition, spirits such as rabb and dëm create problems by inhabiting human bodies and causing infertility or mental illness (Zemplini 1968). Many healers make protective amulets using Koranic verses that will be worn on the body. Other remedies include ingesting medicine through food or drink, or bathing in medicines said to have protective properties. Although preventative actions differ by practitioner, almost all healers recognize the importance of preventative and protective medicines against such beings. Senegalese debate whether "good Muslims" believe in spirits that stem from pre-Islamic cultural beliefs. Some argue that belief in God is sufficient and a faithful Muslim does not wear amulets and other protective charms. Yet many Senegalese who forgo these kinds of preventative behaviors acknowledge that malevolent forces exist, but they choose to rely on God instead of the protective power of amulets manufactured by human hands.

In the course of conversations about my research, I often asked men and women to describe the significant differences between "Western medicine" and "Wolof medicine." Villagers and town residents frequently responded that biomedicine was less useful than local therapies as it is limited to expensive curative care and offers few modes of prevention. In contrast, Islam and local mystical knowledge systems lend themselves to seeking blessings and protection for all kinds of ventures and activities. Some specialists offer protection for travelers, luck for students passing exams, and safe passage to fishermen who spend days at sea or drivers who spend long hours on unsafe highways. People describe these protective measures with a nonchalance that demonstrates their banality; they are part of what "everybody knows and does." According to Wolof common sense, because evil eye and tongue; jealous neighbors, friends, and family; witches, sorcerers, and spirits are all part of the social world, individuals should take necessary precautions to protect themselves. People with special needs (a desire to travel overseas, for example) might seek out renowned healers with a reputation for bringing about desired ends, or to obtain special protection such as a remedy called *tuul* for rendering one's body impenetrable to metal weapons such as knives, machetes, and bullets.

While there is a range of investment of time, energy, and money in these kinds of preventative strategies, I found widespread agreement that they are necessary and effective. Infants and small children are thought to be particularly vulnerable; one would be hard pressed to find a child that did not have one or several amulets on her wrists, ankles, and neck. Merchants who work in large markets or individuals who have steady social contact with strangers expose themselves to tremendous chance of misfortune, and they often take additional precautions to protect themselves. Many Senegalese would argue that a minimum of protection is necessary, and those who choose not to protect themselves are at great risk.

In addition to mystical knowledge, many people seek Islamic cures for more naturalistic pathologies. There are seemingly endless interpretations of how Muslims can employ Islamic knowledge and practice for protection and to reduce vulnerability to disease. In the words of one Pikine resident, "Islam has healing. There are verses if you drink them or bathe with them there will be something in you that is healed.[2] You have a fever and mocc it with the Koran and it gets better, or an abscess and they say a prayer over you and it gets better. Whatever pain you have, there is something in the Koran to make it better." In addition to knowledge of Islam and how it can be used for healing, women have extensive knowledge of different Islamic practitioners and their medical specialties. Women's perceptions of the efficacy of sëriñ contrast with the litany of complaints made about the incompetence of health post nurses and the staff at the Saint Louis hospital. Although there are charlatans and men who pass themselves off as sëriñ to deceive people and make money, sëriñ are usually portrayed as knowledgeable and pious older men who are willing to use their extensive knowledge of Islam to help others.

The expense of biomedical care was a common complaint among poor women, but the quest for a cure can outweigh concerns about cost, provided that the patient and her family can obtain money for treatment. One advantage of frequenting the sëriñ is the ability to pay in kind with clothing or other goods, which allows many people to get treatment when they have no cash to pay for care elsewhere. Women recognize that Wolof medicine can be quite expensive, but they noted the greater flexibility in type of payment and timing of payment than at a clinic or the hospital. There is often a willingness to pay exorbitant fees in the hope that an effective treatment will be found: "Even if you go to the sëriñ you are still going to pay. And there are some who are more expensive than the hospital. If you are sick with rabb (spirits), if you go to the sëriñ you are going to spend more than you would at the hospital. Sometimes the sëriñ can be very expensive." Although cost can be an impediment, therapeutic itineraries reflect the intersection of considerations of cost, efficacy, and accessibility (both geographic and social). Most illness episodes follow the pattern of lambatu, going back and forth between different kinds of practitioners until one finds a remedy or simply gives up.

Waiting for God

For many Senegalese, human action is essential to overcoming illness, but the search for a cure is above all the search for a remedy through which God's healing power can operate. Patients and their families may expend tremendous effort in the search for effective therapy, but this quest is grounded in the conviction that God ultimately determines the outcome of all illnesses. Strategies like lambatu require a large degree of initiative and perseverance on the part of caretakers. Women emphasize that faith in God is still fundamental to all health action: "You still have to pray to God, because God is the only one who knows where the healing is. You mix everything up. You go to the doctor if the dispensary is no good, you go to the hospital and if it doesn't get better you go to the sëriñ who can give you garabu wolof until God makes you better. Whatever God does, people are just preparing the ground for it." The opposite of actively searching for relief from affliction is "waiting for God." In one woman's words, "Some people are sick and they have no money. They wait for God to change their situation in one way or another." This response to misfortune and ill health was described in many of the Pikine focus group discussions: "Those who are sick wait for God to make them better."

Regardless of how one seeks solutions, prayer and faith are part of all therapeutic strategies. Most people assert that they will become better only with God's help no matter what kind of remedy they try. Relinquishing a medical problem to a higher power is a logical response to a baffling illness or to a lack of means for pursuing treatment. Leaving things "in God's hands" is a strategy that most women associate with having exhausted all other options. "Everyone has limits to their means. You could be at home and you don't have any money to go to the dispensary, you don't have any money for the hospital. You are at home trying to heal yourself with certain cures until God makes you well." Even when one is unable to pursue medical treatment or when remedies have proven ineffective, women believe their fate is in God's hands. When all else fails, maintaining faith in God and performing daily religious practice serve as a means of coping with illness.

However powerful one's faith in God, medical personnel were unimpressed with people who were too quick to relinquish their agency instead of pursuing medical treatment. The village health worker Khadi criticized this passivity with a Wolof proverb that argues "even if you believe in God, you still have to till your field."[3] One nurse's aide in Pikine expressed her frustration with patients who give up too easily: "When people are sick they buy medicines one time and then if they feel better they don't do anything . . . or they say they are tired of buying aspirin and they just want to leave it in God's hands. With that, God might make them better, or something else could come of it. Sometimes you put on your shoes and you go to check up on them to see if they are better. Me, if I sell you medicine I am going to go see if you are better or not. If you aren't better I will tell you to go back to the dispensary." Although this aide does not address the financial obstacles that prevent people from seeking biomedical care, she suggests that they often become discouraged and abandon treatment before they have truly exhausted their available options. In her mind waiting for God is a legitimate strategy, but only after pushing one's options to the limits.

There are many competing ideas about the body, health, disease, risk, and prevention that circulate in the Saint Louis region (and throughout Senegal) by way of education campaigns, print media, radio, television, and in everyday conversations. Men and women's comprehension of particular diseases and health issues are the outcome of ongoing dialogues among multiple sources of information: the public health sector, popular culture and media, Wolof notions of prevention and cure, and Islamic discourses. Women have many strategies for prevention and for resolving illness episodes, but most would fall into the overarching strategy of lambatu, which means trying everything possible and going back and forth between a variety of treatments and practitioners.

The ways that medical professionals in Saint Louis, from health hut workers to physicians, misread the health actions and health knowledge of villagers and town residents are problematic if not surprising. Several ethnocentric assertions are embedded within the overarching claim that Senegalese must learn to become responsible for their health. Medical personnel frequently recognize only health action that brings patients to biomedical facilities, which leads them to conclude that patients are passive, that they fail to respond early on to illness, that they don't believe in prevention, or that they simply don't understand the benefits of biomedicine. Tacit acknowledgment that user fees and time constraints limit women's ability to frequent government clinics does little to modify the complaints that nurses and health hut workers make about the public's complacence in the face of disease. All of the medical staff that I came to know during my research are fluent in the diverse knowledge frameworks that inform health practice, and yet their biomedical training and professional status often provoked harsh judgments about local patterns of health seeking.

In spite of biomedicine's dominance in Senegal's development circles and public health discourses, women's experiences indicate that biomedicine does not lend itself to addressing many of their ailments. Biomedicine and biomedical professionals often come up short in meeting expectations of therapeutic encounters and resolving illness. Islam offers seemingly countless means of seeking protection and health in the form of prayer, amulets, alms, pilgrimages, and blessings. These proactive strategies available through Islam and Wolof ethnomedicine contrast with the very limited biomedical views of what constitutes prevention. Women's concerns about health and their struggles to obtain medical care refute the notion that they do not take responsibility for family health. This idea of personal responsibility, rooted in the individualistic notions of biomedicine, serves to delegitimize the many strategies women employ to reduce vulnerability to illness and to remedy sickness.

In the process of resolving illness, women articulate critiques of the quality and accessibility of different therapies. While Wolof medicine and Islam facilitate preventative and curative health strategies, the reality of social and economic constraints looms large in the minds of Pikine residents. Decision making about treatment takes place within a context where cash is often an important determinant of access to health care. Beyond the recognition of structural obstacles is the conviction that God is the medicine for everything, and that all people with illnesses are ultimately "waiting for God." Decision making and health care strategies are the result of the intersecting influences of one's economic situation, cultural knowledge frameworks, and the availability of medical resources.

The following chapters move the discussion of medical pluralism and knowledge frameworks to an examination of how power influences health decisions. As in town, villagers are inclined to make use of a range of medical traditions, particularly mystical knowledge based in mastery of Islamic texts. Rather than conceive of biomedicine, Islam, and local therapeutic traditions as bounded or mutually exclusive health systems, patients and their families easily navigate among different conceptions of prevention, etiology, and treatment and employ many health strategies simultaneously. Therapeutic choices stem from a wide variety of contingent factors, from the availability of different therapies or practitioners, perceptions of their efficacy and appropriateness for a particular complaint, to cost and physical proximity. In chapters 7 and 8, following specific incidents of sickness allows us to observe how power relations, primarily within households, shape therapeutic decisions and the health actions of various family members. The social relations in highly stratified Wolof families produce different gradients of inequality related to age, gender, and generation, and these dynamics play a significant role during illness episodes.

7

Gender, Social Hierarchy, and Health Practice

This chapter moves from a discussion of knowledge frameworks that inform health action to the daily health dilemmas confronting families in Ganjool. My insight into the lived realities of staying well and responding to disease in rural Senegal emerged during the eight months that I lived in Daru-Mumbaay in 1999. I had been a frequent visitor there since my debut in the village in 1993 as one of the first tubaabs (westerners) to spend any time living, socializing, and conducting research in the village, as opposed to the frequent sightings of white tourists passing back and forth on land and in tourist boats to visit the national bird park or to picnic at the site where the Senegal River meets the Atlantic Ocean. Before my field research, my visits were brief and my friends would constantly ask when I was going to stay for good, or at least long enough to be more of a resident and less of a visitor. Throughout the sixteen months of my research I was much more of a regular presence, and while living in Saint Louis I made frequent trips for weddings, baptisms, and funerals. The village became my home base near the end of sonsaa season, in May, when I moved from Saint Louis.

During this time I shared in the ordinary happiness and extraordinary sorrows of a community caught in the grip of rural crisis. Most of the young men had left the village for the Gambia, and women, children, and the elderly were learning to adapt to their unsettling absence. The men and women left behind found themselves in a shifting social and physical setting where the collapse of Ganjool's economy was becoming increasingly difficult to overlook. Environmental degradation and the resulting decline of onion farming, the basis of the village's livelihood for the past several decades, meant that economic relations between husbands and wives, and household heads and their dependents, were becoming strained. Though subtle at times, these changes were producing new kinds of conflicts among family members.

Against this backdrop of social, economic, and environmental change I observed how village women were navigating the daily challenges of managing health and sickness. In addition to routine adult and childhood sicknesses, several families in my immediate social network were confronted with fatal illness. This chapter highlights the more routine health actions of mothers caring for young children, and chapter 8 analyzes how families cope with life-threatening afflictions. These illness episodes reveal health knowledge in practice and they illustrate how household composition and family power relations influence treatment decisions and illness outcomes. In spite of the vast repertoire of treatment options available through Islam, Wolof medicine, and biomedicine, gendered power and authority in families and households often imposed stark limits on women's health action.

The Politics of Gender and Household

Most of what I learned about household and gender politics came from my three closest female friends, Khadi, Faatu, and Jeynaba, who lived in a compound immediately behind my household in Ngeyeen. Faatu, the ringleader of this group, had been widowed in her late thirties when her husband died of cancer, leaving her with a half-dozen young children. In the normal scheme of things she would have married one of her husband's brothers but there were no suitable candidates. Her deceased husband's sister, wanting to make sure that her nieces and nephews were looked after, brought Faatu into her own household by marrying her off to her own husband. This was an unusual situation, but in essence it followed the leviratic practice of widows marrying the sibling of their dead husband. Faatu found herself in her early forties married to a man twenty years her senior. He couldn't believe his good fortune at being awarded a second wife through no effort of his own. Even after her remarriage, Faatu and her children stayed in her original room and her new husband would alternate nights between his senior wife in the main household and Faatu in her small bedroom in the Gey compound.

Jeynaba's husband and Faatu's first husband were brothers, which explained how the two women ended up living in the same compound. Jeynaba had been the village beauty of her day, and the son of a well-established village family with deep roots in Ganjool courted her and they got married when she was in her early twenties. She never spoke of the early days of their courtship, but by the time I met her she was suffering in a difficult marriage. Her husband was away much of the time, and he frequently neglected to give her the daily food allowance for marketing. She was painfully thin and struggling to take care of five children under the age of eight with little assistance from her husband.

Khadi, one of the village health hut workers, was related to Faatu and to Jeynaba's husband. Her father was also a Gey, but he had left the village for

Pikine several decades earlier. Khadi grew up in Saint Louis, but the village chief recruited her to return to the village when he was asked to select several women to serve as the village health workers. She agreed to come and she brought her young daughter with her. Her husband, a tailor, was living and working in a town near Dakar, and he was in the process of building a house for his growing family. Khadi always said that she was just biding her time in Ganjool, and as soon as her husband was finished with the house she would leave the health hut and move to Thiès. She resided in an empty room in the extended Gey compound though she ate most of her meals at the home of her paternal uncle a few households away.

My three friends lived, cooked, ate, and socialized together in a small compound that consisted of five or six cement rooms arranged in a square around a large open sandy area with several mature shade trees. Faatu's husband went back and forth between the main house and Faatu's room, and Jeynaba's husband was frequently working or off socializing with his peers, so their courtyard was a predominately female space filled with women and small children. Every night after the evening meal, Faatu and Jeynaba would bring out their plastic mats and we would lounge under the stars discussing the day's events. Faatu was constantly fiddling with her FM radio, trying get a signal strong enough to hear the news in Wolof. Jeynaba was in charge of the charcoal brazier and brewing the three rounds of tea that accompany all real socializing in urban and rural Senegal. I was responsible for hours of entertainment by asking questions that were completely obvious to everyone else, and for keeping my three friends busy trying to socialize me into the proper ways of womanhood, wifedom, and general personhood in the village.

This cohort of women in their thirties and forties was relatively senior in Ngeyeen. Newly married women are typically in their early twenties, and most become residents of their husband's compounds. Young men and women usually get married when the potential groom has saved enough cash to pay the brideprice of the young woman he has been courting.[1] Most men accrue enough cash to marry between the ages of twenty and twenty-five, while most brides are between the ages of sixteen and twenty. Residence patterns are patrilocal; the new wife will join her husband's family, residing with him in a room that he builds for her in his father's compound. In most households there are two or three senior wives (co-wives of the senior patriarch) and then a cohort of junior wives who have joined the household by marrying the patriarch's sons.

For an indeterminate amount of time the senior male is financially responsible for all of these family members, although his adult sons contribute to the household expenses, and they are responsible for the clothing and other expenses of their wives and children. As the father ages, his sons increasingly surpass his earning power and take on additional financial responsibilities for the household. Junior males strive to acquire enough financial power to branch off from their father's household and establish their own. The junior male is then responsible for his own nuclear family and will often marry another woman. Eventually his sons will be old enough to marry and bring their wives to the household. This financial independence from one's father does not require physically leaving his compound, so there can be two separate extended families living in one compound, with each taking care of its own meals and expenses.

Extended families eat lunch and dinner together, with cooking responsibilities rotating among the wives. In many cases senior wives have adult daughters old enough to take their place in the cooking rotation. In Khadi's uncle's household, where she ate lunch every day, there was a rotation of five women; each woman would take a two-day turn of cooking for the entire household of about thirty people, and then have eight days off.

Marital and family relations in Daru-Mumbaay are shaped by Wolof understandings of gender, family, and marriage, and as with most other aspects of daily life these traditions are mediated through interpretations of Islam. As villagers explained, according to the Koran a husband is responsible for the "maintenance" of his wives and children, which includes providing housing, food, clothing, medical care, and education. In exchange for these responsibilities he is the head of the household with absolute authority over his dependants.[2] He is both a *borom kër* (the head or owner of the house) and the *kilifa* (authority figure) of his wives and children. As Jeynaba explains: "When you are married to a man, you must consider him your kilifa because he is one. You must respect him because a kilifa has authority in his house, and everyone in the house obeys him. When he tells you not to go out, you must stay in the house. You must always ask him permission before you go anywhere." In return for this respect and deference, the borom kër takes care of his wives and children. Wives are not required to contribute to household expenses, and women retain control over their own incomes. Women are responsible for bearing and raising children and for performing all of the domestic work involved in running a household. These tasks include marketing, meal preparation, cleaning, laundry, and child care (feeding, bathing, dressing, and disciplining children). In Mumbaay women must also supply the household with water and obtain fuel (in most cases wood) for cooking.[3]

In discussions of a husband's and wife's role and responsibilities, some men insist that a wife should not have to bring any material resources into the home. As my neighbor Yusu Joob explained, "A man with a wife, his first responsibility is to get up in the morning and go out and work for the DQ. He can do different kinds of work, but he has to go out and get the *dépenses* and give it to his wife so she can prepare food for the family.[4] Women work, according to Islam women should work, but whatever they earn is for them. It is for her. Sometimes her husband won't have the DQ and she will help him. No one says

she has to do it. Islam doesn't force them to do it." According to village understandings of the gendered division of labor in Islam, any material assistance that
a woman gives her husband, such as buying her own clothes or contributing to
the food budget, is done voluntarily. While this is technically true, most women
whose husbands are not covering the household expenses feel compelled to
make up the difference with their own earnings.

In spite of Yusu's insistence on men's responsibilities, the decline in farming wages has had an enormous effect on men's ability to provide for their families. Village traditions concerning gender roles in courtship, marriage, and
parenting are currently shifting. Behind the Islamic and Wolof ideal of the male
provider is the reality that many men's "arms can't reach their backs," that is,
they don't have the means to provide for their families without help from their
wives. This contribution to the household can take many forms, but it most
often happens when women supplement the money given to them by their husbands for the DQ. As Shaykh Joob explained, "She might need a dollar for the
meal, but her husband only gives her seventy-five cents, so she takes twenty five
cents of her own money to make up the difference." Most men can't or won't
give their wives the full DQ, which leaves women in the position of having to
make up the shortfall. Women often have to use their own savings for the daily
food expenses, borrow from friends, parents, or a boutique owner, or find some
other means to buy food.

In light of the de facto arrangements in which women's labor contributes
substantially to household food security, many women found it laughable that
their agricultural labor could be considered "voluntary" or that they were not
required to work. As Joynaba explained, "Women can't refuse to farm. The ones
who don't farm . . . they won't have anything. If you need to borrow money
no one will lend it to you." Faatu elaborated on women's need for cash: "If you
work and God blesses you and you have a good harvest, you will have clothes
and jewelry to wear, and your children will have clothes. Because if their fathers
can't do it, you go and get your own clothes and clothes for your children, too.
That's why the women in Ganjool are farming. Sometimes you see men, all
they give their wives is rice. Everything else you have to buy for yourself. If
you see nice beds, if you see wooden armoires here, they are because of the
women. If she has vinyl flooring in her room, she bought it. If she has sheets,
she bought them." There are varying explanations for why men are unable to
support their families. The declining profits from farming are a significant factor. Many husbands wish they could do more for their wives, and the general
assumption was that only a few men actually have more money than they are
willing to spend on the DQ. One husband insisted that it was not negligence but
men's poor earning power that prevents them from taking better care of their
families, "Most of them don't have it, they don't have enough. . . . If they did

their wives wouldn't have to get their own salt. Not even salt." However, women also know that some husbands simply view certain domestic expenses, such as cooking gas, petrol for lamps, matches, and even breakfast foods, as being beyond their responsibility.

One direct challenge to the assertion that men would give their wives more money if they could is the ample evidence that many of them choose instead to spend their money taking on additional wives. Men's selfish behavior was a frequent topic of female conversation. Khadi was brutal in her assessment of men's selfishness on this count: "They wait until they have some money, and then they go and marry a wife. They go and marry wives and they line them up and they can't even take care of them. They aren't taking care of a single one." Building additions to their houses (to add bedrooms for potential wives) and marrying more women are common ways that men will spend their money. Faatu elaborated on Khadi's comments: "If they don't build, they will marry a wife and plop her down in the household. You see some men, they have two or three wives, and you know that they can't even support one. Some of them are looking for second wives; some of them are looking for fourth wives. That is all they do. If men could have their way, they would just go and marry more wives. Cement and wives, that's it. If it is a good year, they will marry another wife." The subject of co-wives always elicits banter and teasing among women and between men and women, but the economic crisis has aggravated latent tensions between husbands and wives over the allocation of household resources. While the DQ and men's desire to increase their symbolic capital by acquiring more wives and more children are traditional sites of conflict, the increasing sense of economic scarcity has prompted acute criticism of men who fail to provide for their families.

Because of these underlying gender conflicts over the allocation of household resources, particularly men's income, reactions to co-wives are varied and complex. For many women having a co-wife decreases their domestic responsibilities and allows them to save money that they otherwise would spend on the household food budget. But women become especially frustrated with men who do not fulfill their financial responsibilities to their families and instead continue to take on additional dependents.

In one of the more memorable research conversations I had in Mumbaay, Faatu, Khadi, Jeynaba, and I debated the pros and cons of having a co-wife, or *wujj*. I was interviewing them about gender roles in marriage, and the subject turned to sharing one's husband with other women. They found my resistance to polygyny to border on the hilarious, although they would frequently taunt each other about the likely arrival of a co-wife if they did not comply with Wolof standards of appropriate wifely behavior. The permanent threat of a co-wife serves as an effective mechanism to ensure that women live up to dominant expectations about their roles as wives and mothers.

In our conversation Faatu explained her resignation and ambivalence on the subject of co-wives:

Here, it isn't even worth it to be against a co-wife, because whether you want one or not you are going to have one. Men think that they have to have more than one wife. There are men who will go and farm and after the harvest they will go out and get themselves another wife and set her down next to you. They can't take care of her. They can't feed her or clothe her. She will be very tired. But any woman will tell you that she doesn't mind. Any woman you ask will tell you that a co-wife is just what she wants. You know why? If the girlfriend is on the outside and he is courting her, she doesn't know how hard it is inside the house. She will just think his house is a fun place. But when he marries her and brings her home, and she is living next to you, she will know what the house is really like. When you are tired, she is tired too. You cook your two days, and then you give her two days to cook. If her DQ isn't enough, she will have to figure out what to do. That is why here, it isn't even worth it to be against wujj. A wujj is one way for you to get a break.

Women often describe men's courtship behavior and wife lust as a mismanagement of limited economic resources, but at the same time there are important advantages of dividing the household labor among several adult women. Women explained that every day they don't cook they are able to save money. One woman in Mumbaay claimed that most women would like to have three co-wives so that the rotation among wives for cooking would be longer. She added that during this free time, "you can do your laundry, take a bath, take care of yourself and your children, and your fields. Because fields is all we have. The ones who don't want a wujj, they aren't farmers. We don't refuse wujj."

Women are resigned to accepting co-wives and see various advantages to dividing the domestic labor with other women, but *doxaan*, or courting, is seen very differently. It is infinitely frustrating for a woman to know that her husband is spending his money (sometimes to the detriment of the household) courting a woman he hopes will become his second, third, or fourth wife. While many women are willing to extend sympathies to men who are unable to fully provide for their wives and children, spending money on courtship was infuriating to my friend Jeynaba: "I have a problem with doxaan, but I would never refuse a wujj. If they are courting, whatever money they have, that is where they are taking it. They might even tell their wives that they have no money, and then go and take the girlfriend money. And that girl might end up marrying someone else, and he will have lost all that money that he spent courting her. And he won't have been doing anything for you in the house. That is why marrying a wife is better than courting." While Jeynaba was speaking of generalities here, everyone knew that her husband had been visiting a young woman in a neighboring village where he was working on a construction site. Rumors were circulating about whether he was serious enough about her to get married, and Jeynaba must have been wondering if she was about to have her first co-wife. Within the following year their courtship fizzled, and he had indeed lost the investment of time and money that he had spent trying to woo her.

The need for a borom kër, a kilifa, access to land, and access to men's income shapes women's understandings of marriage and the concessions they must make to obtain a degree of financial and social security. Regardless of their ability to generate their own income, women are financially dependent on their husbands, so it is always more advantageous when husbands spend their money on the household. In spite of a general consensus that marriage is necessary, desirable, and the normal state of being for adult men and women, and that marriage serves many instrumental needs, my friends' reflections on gender relations and marital tensions also considered the importance of love. In our conversations about co-wives I would explain that my main objection (and a very American one at that) was to the notion that a man could love two women equally. I always argued that there must be a degree of emotional inequality and resulting jealousy in a polygynous marriage. My girlfriends reasoned differently about this, as demonstrated by Jeynaba's assertions about love: "You think that if a person tries to love two people at once, inside his heart there will always be one person that he loves more? If you are a woman, that isn't your problem. You only look at yourself and how you love him. In terms of thinking that he loves her more than you, you don't pay any attention to that . . . you just have to know that if your husband didn't love you, he wouldn't have married you." Jeynaba's comments reveal the logic of tolerance of polygyny, mandated both by Islam and Wolof social norms, but women's daily banter and gossip about conflict between co-wives reveals a much more nuanced consideration of the advantages and dilemmas of sharing a husband. Women constantly tease each other about the potential arrival of a "little sister." There was also much discussion about the honorable way to accept a new wife with one's dignity and honor intact, and much criticism of women who appeared to be jealous of their junior co-wives.

One of women's strategies to ensure the vitality of their marriage it to spend considerable amounts of time and discretionary income maintaining an arsenal of erotic goods. These products are designed to ensure that they remain sexually desirable to their husbands. If men are the *borom kër* (head of the household), then wives are the *borom neg*, or the head of the bedroom (Buggenhagen 2003). Women's sexual power is an important resource and one of few means of negotiating with husbands about large and small household decisions. In town and in the village, women understand that if they keep their husbands happy in the bedroom, they will have a greater ability to influence his decisions and extract other kinds of resources from him. Maintaining one's desirability also serves as insurance against the early arrival of a younger, more attractive co-wife, and that the husband will continue his sexual relationship with each wife once more than one woman is on the scene.

In weekly social gatherings and larger events such as weddings and baptisms, women discuss, compare, buy, and sell the latest styles in incense, lingerie, waist beads, and other erotic items, ensuring a constant circulation of useful tips and products for "keeping your husband caught in your net." This attention to sex and seduction is part of a larger discourse of *mokk pooj*. The Wolof concept of mokk pooj conveys the idea of performing acts of femininity through the womanly arts of cooking, homemaking, personal grooming, and seduction, and it is thought to be the foundation of a solid marital bond. If a woman is having a conflict with her husband, her girlfriends will tell her to get her hair done, put on a perfumed *boubou*, cook her husband's favorite meal, and then take him to bed to restore marital harmony. The court of public opinion often attributes cases of divorce to the failure of women to mokk pooj. Although the strategic deployment of the art of mokk pooj can increase women's leverage over their husbands, it also ensures that women comply with hegemonic gender ideals that emphasize their submission to men.

Gender relations in Mumbaay, and elsewhere in Senegal, are infused with multiple tensions stemming from the necessity of being married and men and women's contradictory aims. In the most overt sense, men have direct material power and moral authority over women. Men are both borom kër and kilifa, and women are dependent on borom kër for shelter and the DQ. Men control women's (and children's) mobility and access to land, and thus their income-generating ability or educational possibilities. Men have the ability to withhold income from their wives or to spend it courting and marrying other women. Regardless of whether they are motivated by love and desire or financial need (or both), women feel religious and cultural pressure to express deference to their husbands and to maintain their sexual interest to preserve marital stability. The perennial threat of additional wives or inadequate financial support works to ensure women's compliance with dominant gender norms.

This nexus of gender relations is shrouded by the overarching Wolof social value of *suutuura*, which loosely translates as privacy or discretion. If a wife complies with standards of suutuura, no one will ever suspect marital strife in her household or discern that her husband has failed to comply with the expectations of a borom kër. Although protecting a husband's reputation with sutuura is a highly valued and respected social act, it also works to disguise the ways that household food security and general household welfare are in many cases a direct result of women's resourcefulness and self-sacrifice in the presence of an errant husband. Direct or public conflict between husbands and wives, though not entirely uncommon, is distasteful in Wolof cultural settings. Women more frequently rely on covert and subtle tactics to extract emotional, sexual, and financial resources from their husbands while maintaining the public image of a stable marriage.

Women's productive and reproductive labor is therefore situated in a social and material context of dependence on men. All involved tacitly understand women's contributions to household material security, yet this contribution remains largely invisible as women strive to convey the appearance of traditional gender roles. One of the most significant determinants of a woman's relative autonomy and economic power is her social position within her marital household. While women in Mumbaay gain little overt power as a result of their economic contributions, they do gain autonomy as they become senior wives who can rely on adult children and co-wives to share the taxing domestic workload. In households where the domestic labor is distributed on a rotational basis among several adult women, each woman has a greater ability to be proactive about her own health and in resolving her children's illness episodes.

Household Composition and Child Health

Through daily conversations with Khadi, Faatu, and Jeynaba, I learned much about the contentious arena of gender relations and household power dynamics. My sense of the daily negotiations between husbands and wives over resources and household decisions was heightened by observing the strategies that women used as they tried to take care of sick children. Jeynaba had a young son under two years old who was chronically ill during my time in Mumbaay. Two other neighbors, Mari Gey and Nabu Faal, were also caring for young children during my field research. Jeynaba was living in a nuclear household with her husband and their five children, but Mari and Nabu were part of multigenerational households where several daughters-in-law had married into the family. The overall composition of each woman's household, and her structural position within the generational hierarchy, had a direct effect on her ability to pursue medical care for her young children. In particular, each woman's relative financial autonomy or her success in negotiating with husbands and in-laws about medical decisions were central to obtaining access to care. Their stories help illustrate how women's health practice reflects the interplay between available health resources and the ability to mobilize them.

Mari Gey lived in a large compound directly facing my own, and she was always curious about my research and why I was always going to the health hut with Khadi. She was in her late thirties and she gave birth to her ninth child when I was living in Saint Louis. Known for her bawdy jokes and raunchy sense of humor, Mari often had her household, friends, and neighbors shaking with laughter as she would regale us with the latest village gossip of old men who were up to no good or women who were plotting to control their husbands. Mari is the third wife of Usseynu Gey, who was Khadi's uncle and the brother of my adopted "aunt" in the village. Usseynu, his three wives, his two married sons and their wives, and many children and grandchildren lived together in his large compound. Usseynu is a farmer who is not wealthy but bears the status of being one of the most senior men in the village. Mari's oldest child, Faama, was eighteen and unmarried at the time of the research. Usseynu's first wife, Nabu, also had adult daughters who were unmarried and were still residing in the household. Two of Nabu's adult sons were married and their wives had also joined the compound. Responsibility for daily marketing and cooking for the household of approximately thirty people rotated among the three senior wives—Nabu, Biti, and Mari—and the two daughters-in-law.

Mari was in good health throughout her pregnancy, and she was quick to resume onion farming after the birth of her daughter Aminata. As described earlier, husbands and wives do not pool their resources in Wolof households, and so Mari had control over her own earnings from farming as well as a portion of the harvest earnings of her two eldest daughters. Most importantly, her eldest daughter, Faama, had taken over her place in the household cooking rotation. Other than farming and taking care of her two youngest children, she had few domestic responsibilities to the larger household. She did farm during son-saa season, but in the off-season I would usually find her relaxing and playing with her daughter on a plastic mat under the large trees in the Gey compound.

Mari's freedom from the time constraints and accompanying fatigue of domestic labor coupled with her income facilitated her ability to devote a significant amount of time and attention to caring for Aminata. She followed her vaccination schedule conscientiously and attended the vaccination days at the health post in Tassinère. Mari also sought a range of preventative and curative therapies for her daughter. Aminata wore the protective amulets given to almost all Wolof infants, and Mari quickly sought treatment at the first signs her daughter had a cold, fever, malaria, or other illness. I accompanied her on one of several trips she made to see a well-known healer in a neighboring village. During these visits she obtained his remedies for teething pains and other common childhood ailments. Mari made use of both Wolof treatments and biomedical care, and she displayed an unusual amount of initiative in protecting her child's health. Aminata was a happy, healthy, well-fed infant, and she did not have any serious illnesses during the time I spent in the village.

Another neighbor and friend, Nabu Faal, is approximately ten years younger than Mari. She and her husband were in their late twenties at the time of the research. Nabu's husband, Assane Joob, is a junior male in his father's household. Nabu married Assane while in her early twenties and joined his father's compound, which consists of his father, his father's two wives and their unmarried children, and Assane's two brothers who are married and have children. Daily marketing and cooking responsibilities rotate among the adult daughters of the patriarch's wives and the three daughters-in-law. The senior male, Nabu's father-in-law, is financially responsible for the household. His adult sons are somewhat financially independent, although only one has been able to *ber kër*, or keep separate houses, which means to break away from the father's house and found his own household.

In 1999 Assane followed many of his peers to the Gambia to work as a migrant fisherman, placing Nabu and their three children, ages six, four, and eight months, in the care of his extended family. Nabu was given a section of her mother-in-law's field to farm, but her well went dry midseason and she had little prospect of making any money on her onion harvest. In her husband's absence she had almost no access to cash, and she was unable to obtain credit in her own name as she had few prospects of repaying any incurred debts. Nabu also had relatively heavy domestic responsibilities caring for her three children and maintaining her place in the household's cooking rotation. In contrast to Mari Gey, Nabu Faal was slower to respond to her infant son's illnesses. She had few resources and no time to make trips to the Tassinère health post or local healers. Instead of taking independent and immediate action at the first sign of illness, Nabu took a wait-and-see approach. When her infant had signs of a cold or fever, she would point this out to Assane's mother and wait for her to determine the course of action. Nabu had to relinquish decisions about when to seek medical intervention to her mother-in-law, as she had no means of paying for Wolof treatments or biomedical care herself.

Although Nabu complained about her husband's absence and her sense of being stranded with her in-laws, some of our neighbors argued that she was relatively well off. In spite of her limited ability to make medical decisions (or any decisions requiring cash), older women in the surrounding compounds were quick to note her naiveté about her position relative to that of other women. "She isn't tired yet," Faatu commented to me. "Wait until her husband has his own house and she is doing all of the work by herself, then she will know what it means to be tired." Although Nabu did not have as much leverage or autonomy as Mari Gey, being part of a large extended family provided a buffer from economic hardship and access to the labor of other adult women, thereby reducing her domestic workload. She had a limited ability to take immediate action when her infant was sick, but her mother-in-law was responsive and allowed Nabu to make trips to the Tassinère dispensary on several occasions.

My friend Jeynaba was thirty at the time of the research, and she had five children ages eleven, eight, six, four, and eighteen months old. Jeynaba's husband, Modu, was in his mid-thirties. His parents were both deceased and he had no older siblings in Mumbaay, so he was the head of his own nuclear household. Jeynaba had no co-wives, which means that she was solely responsible for the marketing, cooking, and domestic labor required to care for her five children. Her eldest daughter, Binta, was eight at the time and provided some assistance with marketing and cooking, but not without close supervision. Jeynaba also tried to farm a small field of onions, but her harvests were pitifully small and barely worth the effort it took to water them.

Jeynaba was in the most unenviable position of the three women described here. Though Modu earned money on a daily basis working as a mason, he was spending most of it courting a woman in a neighboring village who he hoped would become his second wife. He incurred debts with several shopkeepers in the village, and he was notorious for being slow to give Jeynaba her daily market money. Jeynaba was often waiting for the DQ well after the time that other women had finished marketing and begun cooking, which considerably delayed mealtime and often meant that the most desirable fish (or all of the fish) in the village market had already been sold.

Modu was commonly regarded as neglectful, as he often failed to cover even the most basic household expenses. Perhaps even more important to Jeynaba's overall situation, and the most direct source of her fatigue, was living without co-wives to relieve her from the arduous schedule of farming, meal preparation, and child care. As Modu was in charge of his own household, Jeynaba was also without in-laws who might help her financially. Throughout her marriage she exhausted her own savings trying to make ends meet and to provide clothing and adequate food for her children. She and her children were extremely undernourished, and they had very few changes of clothes. She wanted to send her daughter Binta to school, but Modu was reluctant to pay the school fees, and Jeynaba would have been even more fatigued without her labor. Although Jeynaba resented her husband's pursuit of other women, she was somewhat enthusiastic about the prospect of a second wife. The arrival of a second wife would redirect the money her husband was spending on courtship back into the household and there would be another adult woman to share the domestic labor.

The starkest illustration of the plight of Modu's dependents was Jeynaba's youngest child, Musaa, who suffered from chronic malnutrition and at the age of twenty months could not stand or walk. Jeynaba herself, once one of the most beautiful women in the village, has aged considerably in the twelve years she had been married and she was severely underweight and most likely anemic. She had little time or energy for even her youngest child, who experienced several episodes of malaria, diarrhea, and dehydration during my field research period. When he came down with a particularly severe bout of dysentery and malaria, I urged Jeynaba to go to the nurse in Tassinère. Her tired response was, "What am I going to pay with? My front teeth?" Even in the face of Musaa's acute illness she felt she had no recourse to secure support from her husband, and few resources of her own. Sensing that she had no other options I intervened and took them to the dispensary in Tassinère where I paid for the consultation, malaria injections, oral rehydration packets, and antiparasite medicine.

On our way back from the dispensary Jeynaba sought out her husband, who was working that day at a building site in Mumbaay. She gave him a full report of the medical consultation, including the nurse's assessment that Musaa was severely dehydrated and should have received care earlier. This was a relatively public if subdued confrontation designed to humiliate Modu for his negligence, but it seemed to have little effect. In spite of Jeynaba's attempts to make her husband fulfill his financial duties as head of the household, she continued to receive little support from him and had few options for improving her situation. She started a short-lived microbusiness selling roasted peanuts but in the end she did not have enough time to purchase, sort, roast, and sell them.

Jeynaba's prolonged frustration with her domestic situation gradually eroded her ability to be a responsive mother, as she instead exhausted most of her energy for daily survival. Without the presence of co-wives or in-laws to increase the household resources or to serve as a buffer from her husband's neglect, Jeynaba was unable to exert much agency in caring for herself or her children. On a follow-up visit to Mumbaay in 2005 I learned that Musaa had died the previous year. His death was one of millions of "stupid deaths" (Farmer 2005) that would have been easily preventable with adequate food, water, and parental care.

As these cases suggest, women's positions in the household vary and shift throughout the life cycle, but many are dependent on husbands and in-laws to make medical decisions and pay for treatment. Since the implementation of the Bamako Initiative, women in Ganjool have been keenly aware that they will be required to pay consultation fees at the village health hut and at the rural dispensary. These consultation fees, along with transport costs, time, and other opportunity costs pose significant obstacles for poor women. Women in Mumbaay have some ability to maneuver the gendered relations of power in marriage and within multigenerational families, but they are constantly faced with hegemonic discourses that require their submission to the male authority of borom kër and kilifa. The current economic crisis in Ganjool has aggravated latent tensions inherent to the contradictory objectives of husbands and wives in Wolof society. Women pursue adequate financial support from their husbands to take care of themselves and their children, while men often attempt to fulfill only the minimal expectations of "maintenance" so that they can expand their households with more rooms and more wives.

In this context of increasing economic insecurity, household composition and women's social locations in complex family structures are important determinants of vulnerability to illness and access to medical care. Day-to-day management of the illnesses of infants and young children falls largely within the realm of child care performed by mothers and older siblings. Most childhood coughs, fevers, colds, and bouts of diarrhea fall within the domain of sicknesses that can be treated with home remedies, local herbs, and the few pharmaceuticals available at Mumbaay's health hut. Nearly all women collect medicinal leaves and prepare herbal infusions for ailing children, and they seek charms and special prayers from villagers known to have mastered Koranic verses for various ailments. Mothers in Ngeyeen often asked me for doses of the infant chloroquine syrup that I kept on hand when they noticed their children were running a fever. When women have exhausted the remedies that they prepare themselves, they use their own resources to pursue additional therapies or enlist the help of husbands and in-laws to obtain care for their children. In the most advantageous situations, women can rely on their own financial resources and relative autonomy to attain preventative and curative therapies for their children. In the absence of their own resources, women must lobby husbands or in-laws and convince them of the urgency of attending to their children's illnesses. Their success or failure at negotiating for care for their children can mean the difference between life and death.

8

Domestic Disputes and Generational Struggles over Household Health

Throughout my field research I noticed that there were very few occasions to observe men's health practice or their strategies for dealing with illness. Day-to-day management of household illness falls largely within the realm of child care performed by mothers and older siblings, and women and children were the majority of patients at the health hut in Mumbaay and at the health posts in town. Not only are men absent from the largely female spaces of health clinic waiting areas, they are missing from most of the public health and development discourse as well.[1] The majority of education campaigns, particularly those concerning infant and child health, malaria prevention and treatment, and family planning target women. Some messages address men in their role as household decision makers, but there was a notable silence about men's health issues. Other than in HIV/AIDS prevention information that promoted safer sex practices and fidelity, men are largely overlooked by the formal health sector.

This tendency to underestimate men's involvement in health seeking becomes problematic in cases of acute illness. When household sickness requires urgent decisions about therapeutic options, the power of senior men rapidly usurps women's caretaking role. Women lobby their husbands and in-laws to respond quickly in the face of a worsening illness. But they are dependent on men's medical decisions because of the social hierarchy within Wolof households, and also because women usually do not have adequate financial resources or geographic mobility to pursue a course of treatment on their own. When household members disagree about a suitable course of action, the moral authority of the borom kër outweighs the opinions of other family members. Senegal's health system has in large disregarded the social and material importance of men to family health; women have a far greater familiarity with biomedical spaces and are more likely to have social relationships with medical professionals. The family disputes presented in this chapter explore the implications of men's dominant (and often overlooked) role in household health.

In spite of their absence from formal clinical settings, men are very much concerned with protecting themselves from illness and affliction. The three young men in my household were in constant pursuit of mystical protection from malevolent forces, and they would occasionally travel to distant villages to obtain amulets, infusions, and other remedies reputed to reduce vulnerability to witchcraft, sorcery, and misfortune. Their incomes and mobility allowed them to cover significant geographic distances in the pursuit of powerful medicines. In contrast to this ongoing quest for effective Wolof and Islamic protection, they were relatively unconcerned about malaria and other common illnesses. Interviews with villagers about men's health revealed a predominant concern with a constellation of Wolof symptoms that are related to notions of exhaustion and fatigue. *Tooy* is a Wolof illness that suggests depletion, overwork, and bodily weakness that results from long periods of difficult labor. *Tas,* which literally means broken, conveys a similar bodily experience of weariness and chronic tiredness. Many men drink herbal remedies to prevent and treat tooy and tas during the sonsaa season. The difficult physical labor of coaxing red onions out of the depleted sandy soils in Ganjool was manifest in the weary bodies of Mumbaay's farmers throughout the growing season.

My limited access to the realm of men's suffering was punctuated by glimpses into the household politics of acute illness on the few occasions when young men in Ngeyeen became seriously ill during my field research. There were three such events, one involving a young man in my household, and two others in neighboring households. Two of these young men died tragically, and their suffering prompted controversy and family conflict about therapeutic decisions. This chapter tells their stories and analyzes the tensions and negotiations that ensued within their families during their illnesses. These young men's lives illuminate how the changes of the past few decades, and Ganjool's economic decline in particular, converge with preexisting social inequalities in Wolof households.

In each of these illness episodes, an analysis of the politics of health, illness, and death reveals growing fault lines along the lines of gender and generation and how tensions between younger and older men have been exacerbated over the past fifteen years. As economic insecurity continues and young men seek their fortunes by leaving the village, the generational fault line between senior and junior men becomes more readily apparent in conflicts over medical care. These episodes also demonstrate how the unequal distribution of power within a family—both financial power and moral authority—influence the care a patient will receive. These incidents each sparked debate among villagers and members of the larger Ganjool diaspora in the town of

Saint Louis about familial relations and the social process of treatment decisions. These accounts offer another lens through which to view the effects of regional economic shifts and the ways that larger structural forces become embodied as affliction and suffering (Farmer 2005).

The stories told here all involve young men, two of whom were first cousins in their late teens who had dreams of leaving the village. Abdu Joob hoped to one day travel to Italy, while Taslim Gey planned to attend the university in Saint Louis. Both Taslim and Abdu were still farming onions during my time in Mumbaay. The third case involved their older second cousin Dawuda Faal, a man in his mid-thirties who had managed to flee the dismal village economy by working as a merchant in one of the large markets in Dakar.

Taslim Gey was a brilliant eighteen-year-old who walked with a slight limp from a case of polio in childhood. He was extremely popular among his peers for his bright smile and good nature, and he was widely admired for his academic achievements. He was one of only a handful of village youth to earn a high school diploma, and in 1998 he was admitted to Senegal's prestigious Université Gaston Berger in Saint Louis where he was to start classes in late fall. Taslim was the son of one of Daru-Mumbaay's senior patriarchs, Usseynu Gey (the husband of Mari Gey), who had a reputation as both a womanizer and a tightfisted borom kër. As noted in chapter 7, Usseynu Gey oversees an extremely large household consisting of his three wives, their children, two daughters-in-law, and several grandchildren. Taslim was the eldest child of Usseynu's second wife, Biti. Unlike the good-natured first wife, Biti was more likely to challenge Usseynu's authority, and there were many public and private confrontations between the two of them. In one widely recounted story Biti once humiliated Usseynu by serving him and his guests a lunch of *ceeb u jen* (fish and rice) with no fish, telling him that if he only gives fifty cents for the noon meal then that was what fifty cents would get him.

Taslim's life story in many ways serves as a microcosm of the shifting social and economic strategies of Ganjool's youth and the ensuing conflicts they have created. Though Taslim showed an early proclivity for studying at the village school, his father refused to release him from farming. In order for Taslim to attend classes during the day, he had to get up before dawn to water his father's fields and then water them again late into the evening after the school day had ended. In spite of working this double-shift for years, Taslim was a gifted student and he became one of the first from the village to pass the baccalaureate exam that guaranteed him a place in one of Senegal's universities. Usseynu Gey never acknowledged Taslim's outstanding performance in school and seemed reluctant to lose his son's labor for the sake of a university education. Taslim had many dreams for his future, and we often had conversations about his plans to establish an ecotourism resort on Ganjool's pristine beaches overlooking the Atlantic.

My first field note describing Taslim's illness was written in November, several weeks before he was to register at the university in preparation for classes. He was complaining of stomach problems and he soon began drinking a solution of medicinal roots soaked in water, a common Wolof remedy for digestive problems. At this time Taslim was sleeping in the young men's quarters in my household due to a shortage of space at his father's house. Six days after he started the root water, he went with his father to the Saint Louis hospital where he had numerous biomedical exams, including an ultrasound and a scope down his throat to examine his stomach. In the public conversations about his illness people relayed that the biomedical test results were inconclusive and so the family had decided that he had a traditional illness (*feebar u Wolof*), more precisely *ngelaw u seytaane* (an evil wind). His father was planning to take him to a healer in a neighboring village for treatment. At this point in his illness he was experiencing more pain but he was still sleeping at our house.

Four days after his hospital visit in Saint Louis, Taslim moved into Biti's bedroom, a sign that his condition was worsening. In every household in Ngeyeen, people were discussing Taslim's illness and how quickly it seemed to be progressing. At our evening tea drinking sessions, Faatu, Khadi, Jeynaba, and I would discuss the latest news of Taslim's condition and try to guess at what might be causing his rapid decline. Papiis Joob, a young man who had grown up in Dakar and migrated to the United States but was visiting the village at the time, told me confidentially that Taslim most likely had stomach cancer and that there was no effective biomedical treatment. More importantly, no one except Taslim's father knew about the diagnosis, not even Taslim or his mother. I asked Papiis how he knew, and he responded that he had been able to discern the diagnosis from Usseynu Gey's descriptions of the hospital test results. The Gey family had a history of cancer, and Papiis suspected that Taslim was suffering from it as well.

I began a routine of visiting Taslim every day after the noon meal, and I was shocked at his ongoing weight loss. When I asked him if he was taking any medications he told me that he received several prescriptions at the hospital, but they were only painkillers and not drugs that would cure him. For the next ten days Taslim continued to take the palliative medicine and remained secluded in his mother's room. In the following two weeks there was much speculation about Taslim's illness and what, if anything, his family and particularly his father appeared to be doing to resolve it. Many people expressed surprise that his father did not pursue the Wolof treatment for ngelaw u seytaane, as the family had stated that they thought an evil wind was the source of Taslim's affliction. Biti ran herself ragged seeking a plethora of herbal and Islamic remedies for sorcery and witchcraft. She was powerless to influence her husband's decision not to seek additional treatment for her eldest child, and she seemed distraught about his apparent lack of concern or compassion for Taslim.

In one conversation with Khadi Gey (the village health worker), she told me that she was most concerned about Taslim's rapid weight loss. She added that even Biti appeared ill from stress and worry. Khadi concluded that they were going the "traditional route" because Taslim was taking herbal remedies and the family was using prayer and Islamic medicine. In her opinion, Taslim did not have a traditional illness and should have been taken to the hospital. She suspected that the family knew what the illness was, but for some reason they were hiding it.

Although Taslim's father did not reveal the diagnosis, he began telling relatives in Ganjool and in Saint Louis that his son was gravely ill. In most daily conversation the Wolof tendency is to downplay misfortune and serious debility, so this was an unusual admission of illness that furtively conveyed a potentially terminal affliction. Taslim began to receive a stream of visitors from Mumbaay, from other villages in Ganjool, and from relatives in Saint Louis. Most days there was a group of women sitting in the family's yard keeping an informal vigil, a clear indication that most people feared he would not recover from his illness. Although no one explicitly stated that Taslim was dying, this collective social presence and expression of concern for him and his family were indications of the seriousness of his illness.

In the hushed discussions and speculation among relatives, neighbors, and friends, many people argued that Usseynu Gey's behavior was problematic. Taslim had become sick just at the time that he should have been registering for classes and going to new student orientation at the university. Taslim was concerned that he would lose his hard-won place if he didn't register, but his father brushed off these concerns and made it clear that he was not willing to pursue the matter. At this point Papiis, his older cousin, intervened to become Taslim's proxy at the university. Knowing full well that Taslim might not live to attend classes, his older cousin made several trips to the university to register Taslim, reserve his spot in the dorm, and to explain his situation to officials at the university. He returned with all of the necessary forms and documentation and reassured Taslim that he would not lose his enrollment.

Although in some ways Papiis's efforts were an exercise in futility, it was also a gesture of compassion and defiant support that indicated to Taslim that he was respected and cared for by his cousins and peers. Many villagers perceived Taslim's father's inaction as a sign of cruelty and indifference to his son's suffering. They reasoned that only God can determine that a person is going to die, and therefore humans should never act as if death is a foregone conclusion. Accepting and acting upon a terminal biomedical diagnosis is a lack of faith and a premature abandonment of the patient. Though Taslim's father did not say so directly, Taslim understood that his father thought he was going to die and therefore he was not going to pursue any treatment for him or resolve his status at the university. Given the long-standing antagonism between Taslim and his father about his pursuit of an education, his father's management of his illness and lack of concern about his academic future were not out of character. In contrast, his cousin Papiis wanted to show Taslim that he had not given up on his recovery or withdrawn support for him.

Throughout Taslim's illness I was troubled by the secrecy of the diagnosis. After Taslim's death, Usseynu Gey was more forthcoming and we learned that Taslim had been diagnosed with late-stage liver cancer. I was also greatly saddened by Biti's dilemma. Her unflagging efforts to save her son proved fruitless, but they seemed to be a more appropriate and humane response than resigned acceptance of her son's impending death. Many of Taslim's brothers, cousins, and peers rallied around him during the last weeks of his life. Most of the young men in Ngeyeen would make daily visits to Biti's room to see Taslim, and the sight of these young men wiping away tears as they exited her room was a constant reminder of the injustice of his illness and how shaken they were by his sudden demise. Taslim spent the last few weeks of his life sequestered in his mother's bedroom; he died four months after his first symptoms of stomach pain.

Taslim's death was tragic though most likely unpreventable given his late onset of symptoms and the cancer's rapid progression. It seems likely that no treatment, biomedical or otherwise, would have been able to change the course of his illness. Nonetheless, friends, relatives, and neighbors responded very differently to his sickness. Usseynu Gey, long known for being apathetic to his children's illnesses, came off appearing distant and indifferent to his son's suffering and death. In contrast, Taslim's mother, Biti, was willing to expend limitless amounts of effort to save her first-born son. Despite her best efforts, her lack of economic and social power prevented her from successfully challenging her husband's inertia or finding an alternative means to procure medical care for Taslim. Although the three mothers described in chapter 7 had some room to maneuver in the course of treating routine childhood illnesses, in this case the acute and urgent nature of the illness demonstrates the limits of women and junior men's influence over household medical decisions and outcomes.

In the second case of fatal illness, a young woman named Anta was faced with her husband's prolonged illness and premature death in his mid-forties. Dawuda Faal had left Mumbaay for work several years earlier and was a successful merchant in Dakar when he first became ill. After being laid up in the care of cousins and brothers in Dakar for more than a year, Dawuda returned to the joint household he shared with his older brother, Aliun; his brother's wife, Mati; his own wife, Anta; and their respective children. Dawuda had once been the primary financial provider for the household, but he had been unable to work for some time. He and his nuclear family were now financially dependent on Aliun. As the financial head of the household, Aliun Faal was responsible for making decisions about managing Dawuda's care.

Before Dawuda returned to the village, he had received numerous diagnoses and treatments from biomedical and ethnomedical specialists. His illness began with a small growth on his lower back, which one healer attempted to treat by placing a lot of pressure on it with his knee. Dawuda found this to be an extremely painful procedure; when telling the story, he concluded that the healer had dispersed the unknown contents of the lump throughout his body. Dawuda then went to the hospital and the doctors decided to remove the lump, even though they were not sure what it was. After surgery the incision refused to heal, and Dawuda spent several months in bed with the oozing sore. During this period he was extremely fatigued, lost a lot of weight, and could barely get out of bed. After trying many herbal remedies known to promote the "drying up" of a wound, his brothers sought out another healer. They brought in an expert from Thiès (a small town about 70 kilometers from Dakar) who claimed the problem was a worm, which he successfully removed from the wound. The therapy-managing group, in this case Dawuda's cousins and brothers in Dakar, seemed to find this healer credible and they brought him back for several follow-up treatments.

After a year of being sick in Dakar, Dawuda's family decided to move him to Mumbaay in April 1999. His illness went in cycles during which he would experience more or less pain and would lose and gain mobility. On a good day he would be able to get up, bathe himself, and go to the mosque; on a bad day he would be unable to get out of bed. Dawuda's father would visit regularly from his home in a neighboring village, often saying prayers and using other Islamic therapies in an attempt to bring about Dawuda's recovery. After several months, a healer with Islamic expertise and divination skills began to treat Dawuda. He made a diagnosis of sorcery and spoke of a light-skinned woman who was behind the onset of Dawuda's illness; the healer claimed that this woman had been pursuing Dawuda and at one point had given him something dangerous to eat. This healer treated Dawuda for several months but there were no definitive signs of recovery or decline. On several occasions, when they heard Anta's panicked screams and shouting coming from their house, residents of Ngeyeen thought Dawuda had died. Anta had each time taken him for dead, but these early incidents were false alarms. Dawuda's illness went on for many more months until he died just a few weeks before the month of Ramadan in December 1999.

Dawuda's illness lasted about eighteen months, and there were numerous discussions in the village about the treatments he had been given and how his family was coping with his illness. Dawuda himself was much admired for his optimism and his refusal to succumb. In his own recounting of the illness he would laugh about how painful and ridiculous some of the treatments had been. Dawuda approached being sick with a certain equanimity, and he was compared favorably to the neighborhood hypochondriac who got sick at the drop of a hat and spent her time going to Saint Louis for endless medical exams, tests, and prescriptions.[2] Many people reasoned that if Dawuda had been "afraid" of being sick, or too willing to play the sick role, he would have given up on his own health early in the course of his illness.

The social tensions in the Faal household were also a topic of neighborhood conversation and an important dimension of Dawuda's illness. Although Aliun's wife and Dawuda's wife were close relatives (aunt and niece), they did not get along and there were frequent spats between them. Before his illness, Dawuda was considerably wealthier than his older brother, an onion farmer. The three-room house in which they lived had been paid for primarily by Dawuda, and there was undoubtedly jealousy between the two brothers and their wives. Aliun was the default head of household as Dawuda visited the village only occasionally, and his blatant preferential treatment of his own wife and his constant criticism of his sister-in-law exacerbated household conflicts.

After Dawuda's return to the village, Aliun became financially responsible for the entire household. He was notoriously cheap, known for giving only twenty cents (instead of the standard eighty cents or dollar) for the noon meal. Although Aliun could not complain about his new financial burden because of the seriousness of Dawuda's condition, he appeared unsympathetic to his brother's illness. One neighbor commented that Aliun Faal was just waiting for Dawuda to die so that he could expel Dawuda's wife and children from the household. Aliun Faal's most egregious offense happened after a trip to the Gambia in which he collected donations from all of Mumbaay's migrant fisherman to help pay for Dawuda's medical expenses. According to those who donated money, Aliun returned to the village with close to $200. Rather than renewing the search for a healer, Aliun spent this money on rice and other supplies for the household, essentially using the money for Dawuda's medical care to cover his own financial responsibilities. Even worse in the eyes of Ngeyeen residents, Aliun was referred to another healer who claimed that he could cure Dawuda with a treatment that would cost about $100. Aliun was unwilling to spend this much money, so he bought a few medicinal herbs from the healer (a few dollars' worth) and returned home.

Although many villagers were aware of Dawuda's situation, there was no intervention to help him seek additional treatment. Many of his friends and relatives visited him frequently and harshly criticized Aliun Faal in daily conversation. Throughout the final ten months of Dawuda's life, he was mostly bedridden and being cared for by his wife Anta. She was in a situation similar to that of Taslim Gey's mother, Biti: she had no financial or social leverage to influence the outcome of her husband's illness, to determine the treatments he received, or to challenge her brother-in-law's complacency in the face of Dawuda's illness. After Dawuda's death, Anta left Mumbaay with her two children and returned to her home village. It would have been customary for Aliun

Faal to offer to marry her and provide for Dawuda's children (Usseynu Gey, notorious for his pursuit of wives, also offered to make Anta his fourth wife), but this was an offer that would certainly have been refused. Eventually Anta married another of Dawuda's brothers and she now lives in their native village.

In the third illness episode, a member of my household, Abdu Joob, came down with a severe case of malaria shortly after the onion harvest when he had few household responsibilities and more leisure time. Much to his mother's chagrin, Abdu had been making frequent trips to a neighboring village where he would spend several days with his friends and then return to Mumbaay. She expressed her displeasure, but Abdu was an adult (twenty-five years old) and he was not shirking any of his household or agricultural duties. His mother's brother, Usseynu Gey (Taslim's father, and Abdu's kilifa since his own father was deceased), gave him a stern dressing down after one of his trips and forbade him from leaving Mumbaay. Abdu was nonplussed about the warning, which seemed to be merely an occasion to humiliate and embarrass him.

The following week Abdu made another trip to visit his friends, and upon his return his uncle Usseynu confronted him forcefully in the yard that adjoins the two households. I did not observe the exchange, but a neighbor told me that the most shocking thing that Usseynu Gey said in the midst of the dispute was, "*Yalla nga dey*" (may God kill you). Given the widespread understanding that the spoken word has the power to affect material conditions and events, this was an aggressive attack. Another friend who relayed the story said that he just couldn't believe Usseynu Gey had used these words, and that it had given him chills just hearing it. The following evening Abdu was not feeling well, and the next day he collapsed while walking across our yard. His half-brother Papiis Joob decided to take him to the hospital immediately. When Usseynu Gey learned of the situation, he declared that under no circumstances should Abdu be taken to the hospital. His uncle asserted that Abdu was probably exaggerating his illness and should just be given some pills.

Papiis blatantly ignored his uncle and flagged a taxi to go to Saint Louis. Papiis's ability to take immediate action was related to several factors. As a young man who had migrated to the United States he had acquired symbolic and material capital well beyond most young men of his age (mid-thirties). His permanent residence outside of the village combined with his social capital also meant that he was more willing and able to transgress local norms of deference to patriarchal authority. Normally Abdu's mother would have been responsible for determining the therapeutic response to Abdu's collapse. It is impossible to know what she would have done had Papiis not been there, especially as she is heavily in debt and would have had no cash to pay for biomedical treatment. As a middle-aged widow she is responsible for her own household, but under normal circumstances she would have turned to her brother Usseynu for financial assistance as the eldest male family member and her defacto kilifa.

Abdu was admitted to the hospital in Saint Louis and put on a chloroquine drip. The doctors told Papiis that his condition was quite serious and that delaying his hospitalization would have aggravated his case of malaria. Papiis covered Abdu's medical expenses, which on the first day amounted to US $20 plus another $25 for renting the taxi that took him to the hospital. By the time Abdu was released from the hospital, Papiis had spent about $60, a relatively small sum for him as an overseas emigrant but likely the difference between life and death for Abdu. His mother would not have had the money to pay for treatment, and the next closest relative, his maternal uncle, was clearly unwilling to participate financially or otherwise.

In a sign of protest, Papiis refused to greet his uncle or inform him of Abdu's status when he returned from Saint Louis the night of Abdu's hospitalization. Several women from Usseynu's household, including his first wife, Nabu, came over to ask after Abdu. The general consensus of almost all concerned was that "*lammiñ baaxul.*" This literally means that "the tongue is bad" but implies that speech is dangerous and that Usseynu Gey should not have made his vengeful statement. Papiis had clearly gone against the authority of an elder by taking Abdu to the hospital, but he saved his life and there was a strong community consensus that he did the right thing. Given the escalating conflict between Abdu, his mother, and his uncle about how he was spending his free time, the incident reflects the increasingly acute generational conflict over young men's autonomy.

These illness episodes demonstrate the ways that household social processes influence the management of disease. In each case, medical care was denied or cut short by the adult male family member (kilifa) responsible for making medical decisions. In Taslim's case, he had worked on his father's onion fields throughout high school, but he was about to leave the village to pursue a university education in spite of his father's tenuous support of his educational goals. His father alone was privy to Taslim's terminal diagnosis, and he abruptly stopped pursuing treatment, much to the chagrin of Taslim's mother, siblings, and more distant relatives and neighbors. Villagers spoke poorly of Taslim's father, accusing him of being unfeeling in the face of his son's decline and recalcitrant about paying for his care.

Dawuda had a contentious relationship with his older brother, who was known to be jealous of his financial success as a merchant while he continued to struggle as a farmer. Long considered stingy by nearly everyone in the village, when he became responsible for Dawuda's medical treatment he failed to provide him with adequate care. Even worse, he used money that had been donated for Dawuda's care to cover his own household responsibilities. Like Taslim's mother, Dawuda's wife Anta had little leverage over the kilifa to persuade him to pursue a more proactive course of treatment for Dawuda.

In the third case, a potentially fatal outcome was avoided because Abdu's older brother had the financial resources and audacity to disobey the kilifa's assertion that no care should be sought after Abdu collapsed. Abdu's kilifa, in this case his maternal uncle, had no justification for denying him care other than his claim that Abdu was defying his elders (primarily his mother) by leaving the village without permission. The uncle's refusal to provide him with medical care came shortly after a public confrontation between the two in which the uncle had cursed him.

While the economic decline of the region over the past twenty years is not the direct cause of these illness outcomes, it has exacerbated latent social tensions, particularly over household resources and household labor. There are multifaceted struggles to control young men's labor and mobility. The older generation has a vested interest in maintaining their access to young men's labor for as long as possible, while young men are increasingly pursuing alternative economic strategies that release them from the authority of senior men at an earlier age. In all three stories, the patients could be seen to be challenging the moral influence or social position of the household kilifa either by direct defiance or the withdrawal of their productive labor. Each patient's loyalty to the family or future potential to contribute to the household economy was in question, at least in the minds of the key decision maker. These generational tensions seeped into the therapeutic arena when young men became ill and senior men asserted their authority by denying them access to treatment.

In each household there was conflict among the immediate family about how to manage the illness at hand. While different household members might have access to health-enabling resources, such as time and income, hierarchies of age and gender constrain decision-making power. Decisions about the care to be sought (if any), how much money should be spent, and who should pay are all subject to negotiation, albeit little actual negotiation occurs when the primary decision maker has made up his mind. Unlike the therapy-managing groups made famous in Janzen's 1978 work on southern Africa, in this sociocultural setting the power to determine the course of treatment often resides in a single person, the household kilifa. Though senior men are losing control of young men's productive labor, the ability to deny them access to medical care or to end their medical treatment is a potent reminder of their remaining social power. The Wolof cultural script regarding deference to the kilifa's moral authority makes it difficult for dependents to challenge his medical decisions.

These stories situate the suffering of young men in Mumbaay within a larger context of structural violence affecting the Ganjool region and much of Senegal (Farmer 2004). These young men are embedded within larger social, economic, and political structures, and they are subject to the hierarchical constraints of Wolof social systems as they navigate their changing life options (A. Diop 1985; Gamble 1957). The ways that macro- and microlevel forces affect the therapeutic process and vulnerability to disease, and how patients experience these processes, is largely unanalyzed and unacknowledged in the neoliberal primary health care agenda (Janes 2004). Assumptions about the capacity of individuals to chart a rational course of action in the face of illness overlook the multiple agendas at play in the "serious games" of material production and social reproduction in these threatened communities (Ortner 2006). In spite of their dreams of escape and hopes for a brighter future, the young men in this community can fall prey to the ancien regime of senior male power and privilege.

In addition to these generational fault lines, the experiences of Mari, Nabu, and Jaari described in chapter 6 are indications of how ongoing economic crisis aggravates existing household tensions between women and men. Wolof society has always been highly stratified by age, caste, gender, and generation, so there is no idyllic past in which families lived together without conflict. Nonetheless, the environmental and economic changes of the past two decades have heightened the divergent agendas of men and women and senior men and their male dependents. Women are finding it increasingly difficult to secure adequate financial support from their borom kër, and men themselves describe frustration with their meager economic options and inability to provide for their families. The numerous ways that women supplement household incomes, particularly food security, have done little to affect the balance of power between husbands and wives. Gender hierarchies, which are reinforced by Wolof social norms and appeals to Islam, remain firmly in place. Women encounter these hierarchies when family illness requires therapies beyond their economic or geographic reach, and they must secure the support of their husbands or in-laws to resolve an illness episode.

The story of Ganjool's junior men has been one of relative success, as more and more young men have successfully extricated themselves from the farming economy and pursued their livelihoods as migrant fishermen. Occasionally, junior men will become small-scale merchants and traders, but by far the favored exit strategy is migrating to the Gambia to work as crew on a fishing boat. Many young men find themselves able to become the captain of their own boat after several campaigns as hired boat hands. During my visit to Mumbaay in 2006, several new home sites were under construction in Ngeyeen; young migrant fishermen were building these homes for their new wives. The rapid exit of these young men from the farming economy has threatened the generational dominance of senior men who control access to onion fields and traditionally benefit from the labor of their adult sons. Bouts of acute illness are one of the few occasions where senior kilifa can exercise absolute authority over household decisions about medical care.

These social fault lines and their implications for health practice and therapeutic decision making raise significant challenges to the state's rhetoric of patient responsibility and participatory health action. The notion of "responsi-bilization" and accompanying efforts to promote biomedical prevention and curative behavior belie the complexity of household illness management. Education campaigns to change health behavior are consistently targeted at women, who are assumed to be largely responsible for infant care and respond-ing to childhood illnesses. This is true, but only to a point. While health officials encourage women to be proactive when it comes to preventative medicine and to respond quickly to early signs of illness, many women have very little ability to challenge the power relations that exclude them from household decision-making processes. Efforts at health development fail to acknowledge the ways that women's health practice is constrained by their lack of resources (primarily time and cash) and subject to household authority. Women's best efforts to obtain care for sick family members, as in the cases of Taslim and Dawuda, can be thwarted by kilifa who decide to end the family's efforts to resolve the illness.

The lived realities of sickness and death in Ganjool also challenge state dis-courses that celebrate the new "partnership between state and citizenry" for health promotion and well-being. The household organization of therapeutic decision making, and the extreme social and economic constraints on most social actors, makes it difficult to imagine how this state-citizen partnership would come about. As much of the rural population is barely getting by, most people have neither the time, the ability, nor the inclination to partner with the state on a voluntary basis in the name of community management of the health system. More importantly, inherent to the rhetoric of "partnerships for health" is the assumption that all members of a community, or even of a household, share similar health goals. The cases above demonstrate that health, illness, and decisions about medical treatment are experienced differently along lines of gender, generation, and social relations of inequality. The emergence of state-citizen and even "community" partnerships for health will require far more effort than the national health development plan suggests.

9

Encountering Development in Ganjool

One scalding hot day in the middle of November, I went to the health hut with Khadi to chat and observe her patient consultations. She would often go there in the midmorning and keep the health hut open until it was time for the main meal of the day around 2 P.M. Many mornings were quiet as almost everyone in the village was out watering onions. Business at the health hut would pick up around noon when women came in from the onion fields to do their marketing and prepare lunch. On this particular day, a crowd of women, infants, and small children was gathered around the health hut. Juuf, the nurse in Tassinère, had notified Khadi and Sali earlier in the week that a poliomyelitis vaccination campaign was in progress and that Ganjool's day was Friday. Khadi and Sali had followed his instructions to gather all mothers with children who hadn't been vaccinated against polio. The women started to congregate around 10 A.M. and proceeded to wait for the vaccination team to arrive. There was little shade around the health hut, and women were fanning themselves with their head scarves, fanning their children, and milling around generally trying to stay cool as they waited.

By noon many women simply gave up, especially those whose turn it was to cook that day. Some were able to leave their children with their older siblings, and others had recruited the help of their mothers or mothers-in-law to stay and wait for the vaccination team. I kept asking Khadi if she was sure that she had the day right, and if Juuf had given her any idea of when the team might come. "Yup, it is today for sure. He just said they would be here before lunch. So all we can do is wait." By 1 P.M. Khadi decided that we should walk back to Ngeyeen, so we headed along the main road through the center of the village. We were halfway home when someone in a passing taxi told us that the polio team had arrived in Muid, the next village over, so we went back to the village square to wait with the crowd.

143

Perhaps I should not have been surprised, but when the 4 × 4 truck roared into the village I realized that the polio vaccination visit was literally a military operation. Three men in green fatigues pulled up, a driver and two men riding in the bed of the truck with several coolers of the vaccine. They must have been agents with the *brigade d'hygiène* who were recruited to help with the campaign. The two men jumped off the back of the truck and moved from child to child, squeezing several droplets of the vaccine into each child's mouths. The mothers crowded around the truck, the children wailed in protest, and the agents quickly made their way through the crowd. There was no attempt to explain the nature of the vaccine or to ask any of the mothers if their children had already been vaccinated against polio. Within fifteen minutes all the children present had been given the vaccine and the truck sped off to the next village.

I was mildly perplexed by the whole event: the waiting, the lack of explanation about the vaccine, the quick and dirty approach to protecting the public's health that the vaccination campaign seemed to reveal. No one else seemed bothered by the episode. In fact, this was often how development happened in Ganjool. Outsiders from Saint Louis or beyond would show up with ideas, materials, projects, initiatives, and so forth, they would spend a brief amount of time in the village, and then they would disappear with few lasting traces.

Regardless of Mumbaay's spotty record with past projects, villagers remained hopeful that more development would arrive and resolve some of their daily struggles. This hope persisted despite much evidence to the contrary. Numerous projects have come and gone, and most had produced mixed results at best. In various corners of the village there were artifacts from failed projects. Khadi had several sewing machines tucked away in her room, the only remaining signs of an attempt to create a women's vocational training center in the mid-1990s. My aunt had several farming instruments, including a few backpack sprayers for pesticides, stored away in her pantry. They were leftover tools from an agricultural improvement project that took place in the early 1990s. A few important pieces of infrastructure were in place and operational: the village health hut, a three-room school built by Plan International, a system of small water towers and water faucets brought by an Italian NGO, and a diesel-powered mill.[1] These projects required very little community organization once they were in place, and were less likely to collapse once the development agency left the village to manage the project on its own. The woman's mill was the exception. A woman's cooperative handled the small profits from the mill and used them to purchase fuel and replacement parts. Faatu was the treasurer, and she poured over the mill's books most evenings to make sure that everything was in order.

Several attempts at "health development" took place while I was in Mumbaay. Plan International is by far the most active development agency in

the Ganjool region, and it is responsible for many recent improvements in village infrastructure. The *communauté rurale* (the rural government authority
under whose jurisdiction Mumbaay falls) provided the funds for the village
health hut, and Plan sponsors occasional health seminars that Khadi Geye and
Sali Jah attend to refresh their training. Plan has also donated equipment,
supplies, and pharmaceuticals to the health hut. A French physician based in
Saint Louis, Dr. Huchard, has been involved in promoting different projects in
Ganjool. He often connects philanthropic organizations in France who want to
"do good" in the former colony, and he helped establish a sister city partnership
between Ganjool and a town in France. At the beginning of the school year he
brought school supplies to Mumbaay's students, and he introduced one of the
new community insurance programs to Ganjool residents.

These development initiatives in the village offered an occasion to discern
the interplay of power relations that coalesced around efforts to promote
change. Though the projects had origins in Saint Louis-based organizations or
local government, they were not wholly imposed on villagers, nor were villagers
entirely able to dictate their terms. Instead, development interventions provided an opportunity for the village to capture important resources, and much
like decentralization and participatory management of health structures, they
created sociopolitical spaces where individuals strategize to pursue their own
ends. This chapter examines the process of development as a complex negotiation resulting from the maneuvers of all of the actors involved, from technical
experts to community leaders to intended project beneficiaries (Arce and Long
2000; Long and Long 1992; Peters 2000).

Nutritional Surveillance and Health Talks

Throughout my research, Khadi and Sali were carrying out a nutritional surveillance project at the health hut. They had received nutrition training as part of a
collaborative nutrition initiative sponsored by the Ministry of Health and Plan
International. I learned of the program when Khadi invited me to go to the
health hut with her late in the afternoon one Tuesday, a time that the health hut
would not normally have been open. "We are going to do the baby weighing,"
she said. "You should come along." On our way she explained that all of the
mothers of children under three are organized into groups, each with its own
president. She and Sali tell the president when it is her group's day, and she con-
venes the mothers and children at the health hut at 5 P.M. Once the women are
assembled, Sali and Khadi get out their logbook and all of the children's growth
charts, and the baby weighing begins.

The first session I attended was somewhat chaotic. Children were terrified
of the scale, and they were usually crying before they were taken out of their
mother's arms to be weighed. By the time they were placed on the scale this

crying often became a loud wail, but the children were usually on the scale only a few seconds. Sali and Khadi worked as a team to record the child's weight in the log and then to plot it on the child's growth chart. The growth charts were color coded by age and height: the green zone was okay, the yellow zone meant borderline malnourished, and the red zone meant severely underweight. While these colors are obviously connected to traffic lights, most of the village mothers had never seen a traffic light and could not appreciate the symbolic color coding on the charts. To simplify things, Khadi and Sali just told the women that their kids were "fine" or "not fine," and they pointed out if the child had lost weight since the last session. Most women did not even look at the growth charts, and just nodded when they were told that their children were okay. That day all of the children were in the green zone, though a few were bordering on yellow.

As the baby weighing continued, the group president stirred the nutritional porridge that was simmering on a gas burner. The free samples of high-nutrient porridge were one incentive for attending the nutrition sessions. When the porridge was ready, the president distributed a small sample to each mother in a plastic cup. I later asked Khadi and Sali about it, since there was no real discussion about it at the session. They told me that the porridge was donated by Plan, and mothers could buy it as a nutritional supplement for about fifty cents (US). Each fifty-cent bag is the equivalent of two or three meals for a small child. Khadi told me that they urge women whose children fall in the yellow and red zones to buy the supplement. The nutrition program subsidized the cost of the porridge, but fifty cents was still about half of what some husbands were giving their wives for the DQ. No one purchased the supplement that day, although a few women complained that their free sample was too small.

Once all the children were weighed and fed, Sali launched into the day's *causerie* (health talk). In line with most maternal child health programs, the nutrition program was designed to address women and children's health simultaneously. After each baby-weighing session, the health hut workers would give an educational talk addressing some dimension of women's health. On this day the topic was HIV/AIDS. Sali had several visual aids for her talk, and she began by propping up line drawings of male and female genitalia. This elicited covered mouths and gasps from the group. "Oh my God," chirped Nabu Niang, "there's borom kër!" Unfazed by the crowd's amused discomfort, Sali continued with an explanation of how women get pregnant and she gave a brief overview of sexually transmitted infections (STIs). She showed the group another line drawing of genitalia with lesions, and told them that STIs are very painful and no one could hide the fact they had one—they would have to go for treatment. Sali then used other graphics to demonstrate how HIV is and is not transmitted, and she demonstrated how to use a condom.

Most of Sali's overview was biomedically accurate, although she spoke very quickly and there was little interaction with the group. There were two aspects of her presentation that seemed problematic. First, she made little attempt to actually explain what HIV/AIDS is, why it would be dangerous to women's health, or why they should be concerned about it. Senegal began its HIV/AIDS education campaigns early in the 1990s, and most villagers knew that AIDS had something to do with sex but they were unclear about exactly what it was. One of my neighbors commented that his carrots had AIDS when he gave me a tour of his unspectacular crop that year. AIDS had entered the local lexicon, but not in the way imagined by health campaigners. Even more problematic than the minimal explanation of HIV, Sali ended the session with her own commentary on condoms. "Condoms really aren't that good" she said. "If you use them you won't like them. They are for people who have sex when they aren't married, or who are sleeping with someone else's wife. That doesn't apply to people here, so you don't really need to worry about it." In these few phrases Sali rendered irrelevant any of the new information that the assembled women might have gained from her talk. After going through all of the HIV/AIDS education materials, she ended the causerie with the message that HIV is not really their problem.

It's not surprising that Sali saw little relevance of the HIV/AIDS messages to women's lives in Mumbaay. The women in her audience were married mothers and grandmothers who had very little opportunity to travel beyond the village or to engage in casual sexual encounters. Nonetheless, premarital sex and pregnancy are not unheard of, and there was frequently talk of suspected illicit liaisons. One particularly scandalous incident involved a pair of women's underwear found by a senior man in one of the small neighborhood mosques. Suspicions abounded, but there was never confirmation of which amorous couple had taken advantage of the mosque for their tryst. The increasing importance of migration to Mumbaay's economy, particularly among young men ages fifteen to thirty-five, is another important source of vulnerability to HIV/AIDS. But Sali's uneven message did little to convince women that they should pay attention to the threat of HIV.

The general lack of enthusiasm for Sali's causerie indicates how far removed this kind of biomedical sex education is from the normal domains in which women discuss sex, sex paraphernalia, and eroticism more generally. As in other settings, Wolof cultural norms and social scripts for gender relations and sexuality are not reducible to medical explanations of reproduction and disease transmission (Carillo 2002; Pigg 2005). Talk of sex, particularly in the context of keeping men interested, is not a taboo subject among married women. Sexual capital is of great importance to women, and, as already mentioned, they invest a tremendous amount of effort pursuing the latest styles in erotic undergarments, waist beads, and incense. Women often work for months to create the perfect blend of ingredients for their incense, and then sell their creations to their peers. In the late 1990s hand-crocheted undergarments were the rage—at all of the women's tea-drinking parties I would see women crocheting them, comparing styles, exchanging them, and generally trying to keep up with the latest trends. Any acknowledgment of this vibrant material culture associated with female sexuality, which often reflects women's fears about losing the sexual attentions of their husbands, was completely missing in Sali's attempt to get women thinking about sex and STIs. Her talk provided no entry points or connection to the ways that women normally exchange information about sex, and as a result the content of the message did not resonate with her audience.

If the HIV/AIDS talk failed to situate sex within a cultural context that might have allowed women to integrate the new information in a meaningful way, the main failure of the nutrition program was that it ignored food security as an underlying factor in infant and child health. Mothers were told that their child's weight was "good" or "bad," but there were rarely suggestions about how mothers might improve their child's health. In the cases I observed of borderline or severe malnutrition, Sali and Khadi told the mother she was not feeding her child properly and made feeding suggestions. Working within the responsibilization frame, these sessions were designed to provide mothers with useful information on their infants' health status and to empower them to make better weaning and feeding choices. But as I described in chapter 3, the regularity of household meals is an indication of economic inequality in Mumbaay. At the top of the economic hierarchy were households that could easily afford three meals a day, followed by households that occasionally skip meals but usually eat three times a day. At the bottom were households where meal skipping takes place on a regular if not daily basis. This category applied to nearly twenty-five of the hundred village households.

In the now familiar development trick of turning political and socioeconomic problems into technical problems (Ferguson 1994), the program's emphasis on nutritional information and parental food choices implies that malnutrition reflects ignorance about the connection between food and child development. The surveillance effort assumed that women had adequate food options for their children, and that any signs of malnutrition indicated that the mother was simply making bad choices and should be educated to improve the nutritional quality of her child's meals. But given the constraints many households face in satisfying family food needs, the baby-weighing sessions could do little to make women be more responsible for their infants' nutritional health, or to "empower them with knowledge." Most women were doing the best they could to provide weaned infants with millet porridge and the daily meal of fish and rice. The children not receiving adequate nutrition were the victims of increasing rural poverty, not their mother's poor feeding decisions.[2]

The baby-weighing sessions took place sporadically during my time of residence in Mumbaay, and there were no efforts to evaluate the project's effects on infant malnutrition. Without speculating about the project's success or failure, I can comment on one of the project's instrument effects, that is, the predictable way that the malnutrition initiative transformed village understandings about infant health (Ferguson 1994). On one occasion when I was on my way to a baby-weighing session with Khadi, Abdu Joob, one of the young men in my household, commented, "Oh, you mean you are off to find out who is a good mother and who is not." Mothers were similarly embarrassed when they were admonished for bringing a child who was xiibon, or sickly, to the health hut. Suffused with an emphasis on individual mothers and the choices they make when feeding their infants, the nutrition project worked to depoliticize food security and economic vulnerability. Instead, biomedical discourse of individual responsibility for health was beginning to reshape local understandings of the causes and meaning of mal-nutrition into a moralizing framework. Villagers were coming to accept that mal-nourished children were not due to worsening rural poverty (a frequent topic of conversation since the Diama dam opened), but the result of bad mothering.

Conflicts with Plan International

The nutritional surveillance project reflected the health ministry's focus on child survival and eradicating malnutrition, and it was the only state-sponsored health project with any visibility in Mumbaay. There were other ad hoc projects and plans for future initiatives that came up every few months. Most of these projects were associated with Plan International, and the agency had become a familiar development actor in Ganjool. Although the health hut is technically a govern-ment health structure, Plan saw one of its main tasks as "reinforcing rural health structures and increasing their capacity." Khadi and Sali had the most contact with Plan as they were often invited to trainings and refresher courses, and they were fairly friendly with Assane Juuf, the Plan health coordinator.

In spite of their frequent contact, a conflict arose between Plan International and the village late in my field-research period. Sali told me that she learned of the problem when she attended a health training session organ-ized by Plan. She said that in her sixteen years of working as a village birth atten-dant she was never more embarrassed than on that day. Assane Juuf singled her out as the representative from Mumbaay and announced to the workshop par-ticipants that the villagers of Mumbaay didn't like Plan. He reached this conclu-sion, he told the group, because when Plan employees went to the village to obtain socioeconomic information and to photograph children, they were turned away at every household. The villagers had apparently refused to cooper-ate because they claimed Plan "sells" the photographs of their children to Europeans to make lots of money, none of which is ever spent in the village. This is a logical misreading of child sponsorship programs, but as Sali pointed out when she told me this story, Plan has done many things in the village and their projects are quite visible. The school was the result of a Plan initiative, and Plan had provided all the furnishings and materials for the health hut. Regardless, the Plan enumerators and photographers had unhappily left the village without collecting any information or taking any photos during their last visit.[3] Sali added that after the training session she had tried to go to Plan to pick up some donated medicines and she was told that Mumbaay was no longer receiving their assistance.

On my next trip to Saint Louis I dropped in on the Plan health supervisor and asked him about the conflict. He jokingly told me that "my relatives" were difficult to work with and that Plan had suspended activities with them indefinitely because of their lack of cooperation with the enumerators and photographers. This part of his explanation was consistent with the version I heard from Sali. But even worse, he told me that Plan had paid US $120 to transport a well-known theater troupe to the village to perform skits on various health issues. The village chief had refused to allow the troupe to perform, and they were forced to return to Saint Louis. Juuf was already aggravated with the failed mission of the survey takers, and he said that the wasted expenditure on the theater troupe was the last straw. He reasoned that until the village was ready to collaborate with Plan, there was no sense in prolonging his frustration by continuing to square off against the chief and the other villagers.

When I caught up with Sali again I told her about my conversation with Juuf. She immediately launched into her version of the theater troupe incident, and how she had been caught in the middle between Plan and the village chief, Baay Mamadu Nyang. The day the troupe came, a large SUV arrived in the village square and the new Plan coordinator for Ganjool began asking people where Sali lived. (He was the replacement for a famously unpopular woman named Awa who I was told had been extremely haughty and condescending on all of her trips to Mumbaay. She had alienated the village chief by not asking his permission to work in the village at the start of her employment.) When the new Plan coordinator found Sali's house he introduced himself, and explained that a theater troupe sponsored by Plan would be on its way to perform later that afternoon.

Sali remembered that she had been "lying down sick for eight days" but she got up to bathe, dress, and inform Baay Mamadu. As she passed through the men's *grand place* on her way to his house she told the few men sitting there about the performance. She then headed to the chief's house, and met him coming from the other direction. As she put it, "He had seen the tubaab car, and he likes nothing better than tubaab cars, so he came to see what was happening." She explained that she had just learned that a theater troupe was on its way, sent by Plan, that it would address health topics, and that it was absolutely free for everyone in the village. The first signs of his resistance were apparent when he asked why he hadn't been informed personally and why they were given such short notice. Sali explained that she herself had just found out about the performance.

Within the hour, more SUVs carrying equipment arrived and again they sought out Sali and asked her where they should set up. She directed them to the school ground that is the usual site for village-wide gatherings. The group immediately set up a booming stereo system to alert the villagers that something was happening. According to Sali, the group included "thirty-two tubaabs with cameras and gifts for the *case de santé* (health hut)." Sali says that once the music started, "Baay Mamadu saw me, and he started coming after me, and the other old guys held him back. He started insulting me, swearing at me and saying that I brought all of this here and that I didn't respect him, that I was trying to provoke him. He insulted my mother. I had chills. I couldn't do anything. He is an elder, I am not his equal and he was insulting me. I told him that I would never bring something that he wouldn't approve of. I told him that the moment Plan showed up at my door I came to tell him about it." This heated confrontation went on for some time until Baay Mamadu was finished with Sali and demanded to speak to the Plan coordinator. The coordinator tried to negotiate with the chief for nearly an hour. Many of the elder men came to Sali's defense, assuring the chief that she had notified him immediately upon learning of the event. But Baay Mamadu was adamant that the troupe would not perform. They were sent back to Saint Louis, and Assane Juuf was furious that he had spent Plan's money on an event that never took place. This event touched off the Plan boycott of Mumbaay, which was still in effect when I left the field in December.

This series of conflicts with Plan International, and between Sali Jah and the village chief, stems in part from communication failures, but it also illustrates the tensions between traditional elites and the capacity of new social actors to challenge their authority. The conflict surrounding the theater troupe, which turned into a more personal attack on Sali, demonstrates how her role as a development broker threatens traditional structures of power and decision making. Sali and Khadi were chosen to work at the health hut because they had some schooling and a limited fluency in French. While Khadi travels frequently to visit her husband and children, Sali is always on location and has been favored as a liaison between the village and various donors and projects. She made regular trips to Saint Louis, and she would often return with donations of pharmaceuticals and promises of future assistance. She cultivated a relationship with Dr. Huchard, who provided some medical care to her husband after he became paralyzed by a stroke. When Dr. Huchard arrives to conduct meetings about the school or the health hut, Sali Jah is often the only woman present among the two dozen male elders who have assembled. She not only attends these meetings but she also speaks freely there, and her ability to communicate directly with Huchard in French creates discomfort among the traditional power brokers.

There are three important ways that Sali represents the "other" in Mumbaay: she is Haalpulaar and not Wolof, she is a woman, and she is an outsider who married into the village. For the most part the chief and the senior men accepted her intrusion into the male affairs of managing the health hut finances and negotiating with potential donors about plans for the school. But the unannounced arrival of the theater troupe, complete with a professional sound system (which Baay Mamadu had been known to ban in the village), was more than the chief was willing to tolerate. His adamant refusal served as a reminder that Sali and the Plan delegation could not organize health activities for the village without his consent. Although the village chief misunderstood the role she played in bringing the theater troupe, his reaction reveals his concern about his authority and power being usurped by her relationships with outside agencies.

The village's lack of cooperation with the Plan survey team suggests that Plan International has not explained to villagers how a child-sponsorship agency receives its funding. What the villagers do understand is that they are asked to reveal sensitive information about their household finances and food security, their children are photographed, and the photos are sent to Europeans and Americans. According to Juuf, although Plan raises money through individual sponsorship relationships between Northern donors and Senegalese children, the money is usually spent on village-wide projects (such as the school) that benefit all of the village children. Yet confusion remains on both sides of this sponsorship relationship. Donors often send cash, gifts, and other items to their sponsored child, which creates problems for Plan since not all children will receive these direct gifts. Cash is not usually distributed, although stuffed animals, sports equipment, and other kinds of gifts often are. Rumors about the misuse of the donated funds abounded in Mumbaay when a French couple arrived to visit their "child" in a neighboring village. Although Plan tried to facilitate this visit by sending their staff along as translators, both parties soon realized that the money the sponsors had sent had not been delivered to the child's family. News of this visit spread rapidly throughout Ganjool and produced speculation about what Plan was doing with all of the money that the *correspondants* were sending to their children's families. This incident only increased the villagers' suspicions that Plan was profiting from its relationship with Mumbaay.

Let's Give Birth at the Health Hut

In addition to the school classrooms, plans were in the works to bring additional infrastructure to the village center. The sister-city partnership facilitated by Dr. Huchard was raising money to build several rooms to house the schoolteachers so they would have their own accommodations. (At the time they were each living with a local family.) The other initiative under discussion was Dr. Huchard's plan to construct a wall around the existing case de santé. His idea was that the wall would create a private, enclosed space around the health hut that would transform it into a birthing center. Rather than giving birth at home, women in labor could come to a central location and Khadi and Sali would assist in the delivery there. Although Sali and Khadi took turns working at the health hut, attending births was their primary task as health hut workers. Villagers made use of the health hut sporadically, but nearly every woman in labor would send for Khadi or Sali to check on her progress during childbirth (Khadi was much preferred over Sali among women in Ngeyeen). Whoever arrived at the birth would follow the woman's progress and ensure that everything was proceeding normally. At the first signs of a complicated delivery they would evacuate the woman to the health post in Tassinère.

Sali and Khadi often complained about the inconvenience of home births and the fact that they were always on call. It was also difficult for them to secure the payment they were owed for assisting a birth. The going rate was US $10 for a first birth and around $6 for subsequent births. Since the health hut made very little money from consultation fees, the fees associated with attending births represented the majority of their income. They claimed that it was always challenging to get this payment; at the actual birth things were too chaotic, and immediately after the birth, families were distracted by planning the infant's naming ceremony, which takes place eight days after the birth. Occasionally when we were sitting in the health hut they would call out to a passerby that he or she still owed them money from the recent birth in their household.

Dr. Huchard's idea was to build a tall cement wall to enclose the courtyard surrounding the health hut, and in this way transform the two-room building into a birthing area. One of the rooms in the health hut already had a single bed to accommodate women in labor, but to my knowledge no woman had ever given birth there. Dr. Huchard reasoned that building an enclosed courtyard would afford women enough privacy to be able to labor away from home. I was quite skeptical about this rationale. The health hut is located in the center of the village, directly behind the school and adjacent to the village market and the men's *grand place*. Any woman on her way to give birth at the health hut would have to walk through the most public spaces of the village before arriving there. It would not be an overstatement to say that birth in Wolof culture is a tremendously private, female affair. Most women delay as long as possible before sending for Khadi or Sali because then everyone will know that they are in labor. When I raised the issue of privacy with Sali, she argued that a pregnant woman could be coming to the health hut for all kinds of reasons, and if she passed through the village on her way there no one would know the reason for her visit.

In spite of these potential obstacles to a centralized location for a birth center, Khadi and Sali were enthusiastic about the idea of enclosing the health hut and requiring women to give birth there. "It will be so much easier," remarked Sali. "We won't have to trek all over the village, instead women will have to come to us!" They also thought that it would be easier to collect their fees since most villagers knew that they had to pay a consultation fee before they could receive services at the health hut. When I suggested that women's commitment to discretion might be a major impediment to taking birthing out of the home, Khadi and Sali insisted that if they refused to respond when they were called to women's homes, the laboring women would have no choice but to comply with the new system. They countered that women might actually have *more* privacy at the health hut as they could labor out of the view of their children, co-wives, and other household members. Nonetheless, the initiative seemed more likely to increase the efficiency and convenience of attending births for the health hut workers, and less likely to meet the needs of village women.

For various reasons the plan to create the enclosed courtyard never came to fruition. Khadi joined her husband in Thiès the year after my fieldwork ended, and Sali became preoccupied with her disabled husband's declining health. Sali worked less and less in the health hut and became less invested in helping to facilitate village development projects. In the years since my field research the health hut has gone through various phases of falling into disuse and then opening up again when Sali or the village health committee get inspired to jump-start its operations. Attempts to expand the village's health infrastructure proceeded in fits and starts and then gradually sputtered out.

The Pattern of Development Failures

The different initiatives discussed here are admittedly very small scale development efforts designed to address some of the immediate needs of the villagers in Mumbaay. As such, they did not attempt to disrupt the broader socioeconomic processes that have marginalized the region and crippled its agricultural economy. Since the mid-1980s, when the Senegalese government and the OMVS began publicizing plans to invest in irrigated agriculture in the Waalo region, it has been clear that Ganjool is not part of the state's focus on agricultural improvements. Ganjool has been all but forgotten in national agricultural development plans that have focused on the Middle Valley as the potential bread basket of the nation. Although village politicians maneuver for power and influence on the rural council, there are few mechanisms to demand greater attention from the state or inclusion in regional development schemes. In the absence of large projects funded by the state and multilateral and bilateral agencies, villagers eagerly await small-scale development initiatives regardless of abundant evidence that they produce few if any lasting results.

As in most accounts of botched development, there are many explanations about why attempts to bring about change in Mumbaay so frequently meet with outright resistance or apathy. These failures follow a relatively consistent pattern that ranges from poor conceptualization and implementation to inadequate recognition of social hierarchies and local cultural frameworks. The socioeconomic inequalities among households and families in Mumbaay are largely invisible to project planners, as are the complex social fields in which villagers navigate social strata of age, gender, generation, and to some extent class. Much like the health committees in Saint Louis, development projects open up temporary spaces where villagers compete for access to goods and control. These projects are often co-opted by village elites, or they are cannibalized from the inside for short-term gain.

Dovetailing with the tacit assumptions of health reform and decentralization, most development projects assume that villagers possess enormous latitude to make rational decisions and to act freely to improve their individual circumstances. This misconception ignores the fact that villagers are social beings embedded in social processes, and that their daily practice stems from shared cultural frameworks. The originators of Information, Education, and Communication (IEC) campaigns assume that after women are exposed to educational materials about nutrition or HIV/AIDS, they will immediately incorporate this information into their daily actions. In this model of behavior change, women are assumed to be empty vessels that are ignorant about nutrition, and so they can be filled with appropriate knowledge.

The confrontation between the village chief and Sali Jah illustrates the tensions between traditional forms of power and authority (age, gender, lineage, length of residency in the village) and new kinds of social capital that emerge in the context of development projects (proficiency in French, connections with donor agencies). A scene might have been avoided if the Plan International coordinators had made a more concerted effort to comply with village protocol. But this was not the first time that the chief had asserted his authority vis-à-vis the health hut and health activities. I learned from Khadi that shortly after Plan equipped the new health hut with large wooden tables and benches, the chief had confiscated the furniture for his own use. He now rents out the table and benches to families hosting weddings and baptisms.

Friends and neighbors told me story after story of short-lived development projects. They identified two main obstacles to success: personal greed and lack of literacy and numeracy skills. Most of the projects that had targeted women, particularly income-generation and vocational-training programs, required a degree of financial management and bookkeeping that illiterate women were unable to perform. The success of the women's mill project was that it had offered literacy and numeracy training in Wolof before the mill was built. Over a dozen women attained a minimal level of literacy, and they reported that this is what had made the project a success.

While the anthropological literature on international development has long abandoned the notion of harmonious, tight-knit communities where all members share the same goals and interests, the numerous social divisions that characterize village social life were omnipresent. Conflicts between husbands and wives, rivalries among co-wives, jockeying between senior and junior men, and political jousting among the elder men for positions on the rural council frame the context in which development is supposed to take place. Many of these fault lines remain under the surface in daily interactions, but they can also escalate into private and public confrontations. In light of the increasing economic vulnerability of Ganjool's population, it seems likely that development initiatives will continue to spark tensions and create competition in Mumbaay.

Other development failures stem from implicit (and often incorrect) assumptions about the role of culture in daily life and health practices in the village. Resistance to "progress" is often seen as a barrier to improving health and well-being. Many health professionals believe that this resistance is rooted in cultural ideas about health or a lack of familiarity with biomedicine. Sali and Khadi often blamed local understandings of malaria, and local health practices more generally, for villagers' slow and measured responses to illness. The tacit assumption of the nutritional surveillance program was that ignorance is part of the problem, that is, village mothers were unaware of the connection between adequate nutrition and child health. The project was designed to educate women about this connection, and to encourage them to choose nutritious weaning foods and to purchase the food supplement in cases of borderline or severe malnutrition. The emphasis on educating mothers masks the root of the problem, which is the increasing household food insecurity stemming from broader economic decline.

While "culture" can serve as an explanation for why people don't comply with desired health behavior, in other cases the significance of cultural context is completely overlooked. In Sali's AIDS causerie, she attempted to present information on STIs, AIDS, and condoms with little reference to the ways that women would normally discuss sex. Her health talk could have prompted dialogue, questions, and commentary from her audience if she had presented HIV/AIDS as a potential threat to women's ongoing commitment to *mokk pooj*, that is, to ensure marital harmony by satisfying their husbands sexually. In a similar fashion, the plans to "modernize" birthing practices in the village by creating a maternity ward at the health hut seemed improbable given the emphasis on privacy and discretion during labor and childbirth. The health workers were enthusiastic about this idea not because it would improve birthing outcomes, but because it would make it easier for them to assist births.

Attempts to bring about development were sabotaged by multiple factors, from inherent flaws in their conceptualization to outright resistance or cooptation. Regardless, village residents enthusiastically embrace the idea of development and development projects. "Development" has become the dominant rubric through which villagers hope to remedy their grinding poverty and peripheral status in the region. If development were to happen, villagers reason, they would have a paved road to Saint Louis and their own doctor or nurse to treat their medical problems. Although the rewards of development are elusive, residents of Ganjool continue to lobby rural and urban officials for funding, projects, and infrastructure.

This unbridled enthusiasm for projects rests uneasily alongside a deeper understanding of the profound dilemma facing local farmers. Young men continue to leave the village to fish elsewhere along the Atlantic coast, and villagers approach each onion season with anxiety about their debts and their slim prospects for a successful harvest. Faced with these dire conditions, the continued interest in projects seems misplaced at best; projects temporarily detract attention from a region that seems headed for collapse. The best hope for the residents of Ganjool is to find a new economic niche that will allow them to reverse their cycle of annual debt and to improve household food security. This is a challenge that goes far beyond the capacity of ad hoc projects, and for the indefinite future a reversal of fortune for Ganjool's struggling farmers seems unlikely.

10

Believe in God, but Plow Your Field

When I returned to Senegal in 2002, two and a half years after I finished the bulk of the research for this project, many colleagues and acquaintances in Saint Louis and Ganjool wondered why I had come back. The marriage that brought me to Pikine and Mumbaay had ended, my graduate school years had come to a close, and I was moving on to a new chapter in my professional life. More than a few times I myself wondered what I was doing there. Was I an anthropologist returning to the field, a friend stepping back into the lives of her inner circle, a former in-law seeking closure?

After navigating the gauntlet of social and professional courtesy calls in Saint Louis and Pikine, I finally made it to the village and back into the tight-knit group of women who had befriended me during my research. It was still the peak of the onion season so I found myself following Faatu to her field one morning. I sat on an old scrap of clothing in the shade of an acacia tree while she performed the backbreaking labor of watering her onion plants. She would throw two buckets deep into her well, pull them up by the attached rope in a constant hand-over-hand motion, and walk slowly, emptying the buckets on each side of the narrow path between her rows of onions.

I hadn't told Faatu about my lukewarm reception from some of my acquaintances in Saint Louis, or the surprised and somewhat bemused greetings from others. I hadn't voiced my lingering sadness, or my uncertainty about establishing new connections to a place that I had come to think of as my second home. Yet somehow she knew. "You came back," she offered before I had even begun to speak, "because your heart is heavy. And when your heart is heavy, you take it to the people who care about you so they can help you carry the load." I nodded back at her and we stayed in silence for much of the morning as she continued her rhythmic work, trying to coax life and a livelihood out of the desert.

This book has posed challenges for me as an anthropologist, a writer, a former resident of Saint Louis and Mumbaay, and a friend and in-law to many of the people who appear in these pages. Putting their experiences to paper has been my way of sharing their load, and ensuring that they are not forgotten in the sweeping accounts of devastation and decline in Africa. My commitment to these communities, though a compelling motivation for my own work, is embedded in a larger assertion that their lives matter. Two decades of social and economic change have profoundly affected the life chances of residents of Pikine and Mumbaay, and their stories illustrate the stark consequences of the large-scale processes affecting daily life for Africans throughout the continent.

Social scientists and international development professionals have come to refer to the 1980s as the "lost decade" for Africa given the devastation of structural adjustment lending programs and their effects on a variety of health and development indicators. The irony of this moniker is that the 1980s might have signaled the beginning of the losses, but we have yet to see their end. Aggregate indications of improvement in health and well-being, economic growth, and rising GDPs mask the growing disparities between rich and poor and the realities of Africans living in the "global shadows" (Ferguson 2006). Behind the sensational headlines of AIDS orphans and genocide in Darfur are the less dramatic stories of people for whom barely getting by has become a normal way of life. By offering this account of two communities confronting the daily realities of market-driven economic policies and health reform, my aim has been to draw attention to the less sensational dilemmas facing many Africans in the twenty first century.

My strategy has been to use ethnography to analyze the different kinds of encounters taking place among global health policies, national development strategies, regional and community political structures, and the micropolitics of managing health and illness within urban and rural households. The convergence of health reform with broad-based attempts at restructuring Senegal's government is a historical process contingent upon the actions of specific social agents. Macrolevel development processes and health policies don't merely descend "from above," they are constituted in their enactment, negotiation, and mediation by people in public and private arenas in national and regional spaces (Asher 2009; Gupta and Ferguson 2002). I have tried to capture these processes to demonstrate how they are transformed as they move from hypothetical policies to new operating procedures that must be carried out by a host of social actors with conflicting interests.

One of my primary concerns has been to examine the process of health sector reform carried out throughout the 1990s in Senegal. These reforms were intended to meet specific objectives, including cost recovery for the health system through user fees and the sale of generic essential medicines, and formalizing community participation in the health sector through local health committees.

The negative outcomes of these reforms have become a familiar refrain in the global health literature (Paluzzi 2004; Schoepf et al. 2000; Turshen 1999), and we are reminded that health policies and approaches derived from advanced capitalist economies are often ill-suited to meet people's needs in vastly different settings (Bloom and Standing 2008). Beyond these insights, there has been little attempt to document how global health reforms have shaped therapeutic processes or the arena of health practice in the broadest sense. The Senegalese Ministry of Health implemented these reforms against the backdrop of decentralization of the health sector along with most other areas of government involvement. Taken together, health reform and decentralization marked a significant qualitative shift in the financing, operation, and organization of Senegal's medical districts. The Saint Louis medical district provides one snapshot of the kinds of tensions and conflicts produced as medical district administrators and city officials attempted to navigate this new terrain. Some of the difficulties that I observed were inherent to the context of transition as elected officials and government employees became familiar with the new legal codes and operating procedures.

Regardless of the expected confusion surrounding the new reforms, many of the problems evident in the case of Saint Louis stem directly from the intersection of the reform process with existing social processes and structural inequalities. Social and economic disparities have a long history in Senegal. They have been embedded in a variety of social and political structures, from ethnic caste systems to French colonialism and the hierarchical Sufi orders in which the faithful submit to the moral authority of their shaykhs. In the postindependence period a state run by political elites has rewarded party loyalty and pinned its hopes on the economic development and promise of some regions which neglecting others. Most recently the advance of neoliberal policies has subjected the entire country to the new rules of global capitalism. Unlike past systems of domination, in which some measure of security and well-being were often the reward for submission to higher authorities, there seem to be few if any rewards from this deference to neoliberalism.

Clearly then, the Bamako Initiative and decentralization were not carried out on a blank slate. The most obvious way that health reform compounded existing inequalities is that the municipality of Saint Louis, which was already in a peripheral part of the country, found itself with very few resources to support the health sector. The new mandate for financing social services with municipal resources created a budget crisis for the city. Unresolved disputes between the mayor's office and the medical district were just one sign of the city's economic distress under decentralization. The budget crisis had a direct effect on district operations and the quality of care available at the city health posts. Many of the medical personnel, particularly health post nurses and auxiliary personnel, were extremely demoralized, and their frustration affected their work habits and their interactions with patients. As is often the case, the implementation of cost-recovery strategies reinforced preexisting economic inequalities, and produced "poor medicine for poor people" (Janes et al. 2006; Turshen 1999). Just as the municipality lacked adequate resources to fund the health sector, the poor residents of Pikine and other neighborhoods lacked resources to pay for care. To the extent that the health system was functioning, this is a meaningless outcome for those who have no resources with which to access care (Roberts et al. 2004, 49).

Saint Louis' peripheral position vis-à-vis the state played a role in the difficulties associated with decentralization, but the existing social and political landscape of the city and its neighborhoods were equally important in mediating the impact of the Bamako Initiative on day-to-day health operations. Health committees are the most visible arena in which local elites and neighborhood leaders maneuver to capture political capital and access to health post profits and pharmaceuticals. Although they are touted as the new vehicles for broad-based community participation in the health system, they have become highly politicized. Seats on the committees tend to be won by the "usual suspects" who have little commitment to improving neighborhood health. The general assemblies are structured to encourage the participation of women and youth in the election process and on the committees, but they remain marginal. The underlying irony is that women are the primary targets of health efforts, particularly health education campaigns on maternal and child health, but they continue to be treated as objects to be acted upon rather than subjects whose views and decision-making power would enhance the quality of primary health care (Foley 2001). Despite the current enthusiasm in international development and global health circles for community involvement and partnerships between public and private institutions and civil society, these partnerships are no guarantee of effective or meaningful participation (Janes 2004, 463).

The state's attempt to advance a collective responsibility for health through discourses of partnership with ordinary citizens belies the hierarchical nature of biomedicine and Senegal's government health system. Nurses and state-trained midwives chafed under the mandate to treat their health committees as partners in health. The proposed community management structures were a direct threat to the medical professionals who used to enjoy unrestricted access to pharmaceuticals and the ability to waive consultation fees for friends and family members. While many patients were frustrated by the institutionalization of user fees and generic drug sales, health post nurses felt that their autonomy and prestige as medical personnel were under siege by community members intent on exposing fraud and corruption. Health committees in Saint Louis were convinced that the ongoing health employee union strike was a ploy to circumvent performance evaluations at the district's health posts. These stances of mutual suspicion escalated occasionally, as in the public relations battle between the Pikine head nurse and the health committee treasurer. The savvy head medical officer, Dr. Faal, was able to arbitrate many of these disputes, but the latent structural tensions of the health system continue to undermine community management and widespread participation.

In addition to analyzing how global health trends and national health reform have taken shape in Senegal, I have been equally concerned with the lived experiences of urban and rural families as they attempt to manage risk, vulnerability, and illness. Rather than codify a depiction of Wolof culture, I have focused on key events, conflicts, and personal stories to demonstrate how the lives of real individuals are caught up in the tumultuous changes of the past several decades. The hierarchical nature of Wolof society and the aggravated economic insecurity of the past decades are central to household decision making about illness. In times of illness, urbanites and villagers strategize within the contentious social fields of family and community to mobilize health resources. The therapy-managing group, which is often dominated by the male head of household, wields a tremendous amount of power to determine the course of treatment, and his interests may be at odds with those of other household members.

By looking at the things that people do or don't do when faced with illness, we begin to understand the sharp divide between the logic of market-based medical care and the structural limitations on individuals' health action (Baer, Singer, and Susser 2003; Janes et al. 2006; Pfeiffer and Nichter 2008). Stories about managing sickness, from routine childhood illness to life-threatening diseases, demonstrate how intrahousehold power relations, hierarchies of age and gender, and structural inequalities of class and geography often impede people's health actions. Unequal relations between men and women and juniors and elders often influence who will have access to medical treatment, the kind of treatment they will receive, and which family members will be involved in therapeutic decision making. Mari, Nabu, and Jeynaba had varying abilities to obtain health resources for their children. The dynamics of each woman's household, and her relative position within the family hierarchy, influenced her health decisions. In the cases of the three young men confronted with life-threatening afflictions, we see that the gravity of the illness also influences who becomes responsible for treatment decisions; the autonomy of wives and mothers taking care of family members ends in the face of serious illness episodes that require pursuing health options beyond Mumbaay.

The knowledge frameworks that make up the therapeutic repertoires in play in Saint Louis can be both complementary and conflicting. Rural and urban patients alike follow complicated therapeutic itineraries that they describe as *lambatu*, or going from one option to the next in an attempt to relieve affliction. In spite of ongoing education campaigns for the prevention of malaria, diarrheal disease, HIV/AIDS, and the promotion of birth spacing, biomedicine is far from hegemonic. New medical information and the promotion of new health behaviors are filtered through existing understandings of health and illness. Men and women do not behave like rational, economic actors unencumbered by culture or context as envisioned by health planners and policymakers (Foley 2008). What Senegalese know to be true about health, illness, and medicine is often not what biomedical clinicians want them to know. In spite of admonitions by doctors and nurses to take early action, waiting for God is often the first and only therapeutic option for poor families coping with ill health.

By employing the concept of health practice, I have explored how diverse knowledge frameworks shape local conceptions of health resources without losing sight of the social and material constraints on people's ability to make use of those resources (Meinert 2004; Obrist 2003). Decisions about pursuing medical treatment are contingent upon multiple factors, including the nature of the illness and the proximity of various practitioners. But beyond the variety of therapeutic options, communities in Saint Louis and Ganjool are caught up in regional processes of rapid urbanization and rural agricultural decline. The recent economic downturns have weakened the financial security of individual families at the same time that the state has withdrawn much of its financing for social services. The poor and fragmented quality of biomedical care available in the Saint Louis region is one dimension of the underlying context of health seeking. Stories of acute and fatal illness reflect the broader problems of the region, which is caught up in larger processes that might best be understood as structural violence (Farmer 2004).

If health practice is the result of strategies and maneuvering to take advantage of different kinds of health resources, most health development is an effort to legitimize new health options and to convince people to make use of them. In spite of these attempts to change what people recognize and value as effective health resources, health practice is closely related to social power, and is therefore unlikely to change at the pace desired by health educators (Meinert 2004). One of the chief priorities of the Ministry of Health is to foster effective preventative and curative health actions around malaria, but decades of health education have done little to mobilize a new understanding of Senegal's number one killer. In contrast, hypertension, which dovetails with idealized norms of feminine beauty and social status, has become the affliction du jour in Saint Louis for women aspiring to be drianke. The health hut workers' attempts to promote a biomedical understanding of malnutrition and nutritional supplements had little effect on village women's feeding practices. Women fed their young children from the same bowl as the rest of the family, and the availability of supplements for purchase could not overcome the underlying problem of food insecurity.

Health interventions that counter dominant norms are also likely to be circumvented or flatly rejected. The village chief successfully ended or hampered attempts to promote health development when he thought these activities threatened his authority. The village health-hut-turned-maternity-ward also seemed like a project doomed to fail from the start, as village women had no need for a biomedical space designated for labor and childbirth. Although this new kind of health resource appealed to Khadi and Sali, they would have had a difficult time convincing village woman of its advantages. Cultural frameworks and hierarchical social relations influence the relative success of attempts to change the health landscape. The introduction of medical resources and new health information cannot override the material and social forces that shape health practice.

On a visit to Mumbaay in 2006 I was surprised to find several local improvements that could fall under the category of small-scale development. My former in-laws had a new cement wall enclosure around their compound, and they had paved over their dirt yard and built a thatch porch for shade from the Sahelian sun. Of the three sons living in the household, one was migrating annually to the Gambia to fish, one continued to farm onions, and the eldest was making a living as a middleman buying and transporting onions and other produce and selling them in other regions of Senegal.[1] This diversified economic strategy provided them with enough income to invest in household infrastructure and remain relatively debt-free. At the center of the village stood a new agriculture microcredit office, where villagers with collateral (i.e., men who owned land) could receive low-interest loans at the start of the agricultural season to purchase inputs and other agricultural commodities. I marveled aloud at the number of changes to the village and the neighborhood in the course of a year, and my friend Awa responded, "Well, you know, sometimes progress can sneak up and take you by surprise."

In thinking about her comment, I was struck by the defiant resilience of survival, and the celebration of something resembling progress, in the face of unimaginably bad odds. Forgotten by the state, skipped over by the integrating processes of globalization, people in Pikine and Mumbaay persevere. They do so in the absence of any indication that their economic marginalization will be addressed by the state or that development will arrive once and for all and alleviate the worst of their hardships. This survival doesn't come without causalities. Musaa's death in 2005, and the deaths of so many others, offers abundant evidence of the ways that structural inequalities become embodied as illness and fatality in places like Ganjool. Nonetheless, every morning villagers get up and do what needs to be done, believing in God and plowing their fields.

NOTES

CHAPTER 2   A BRIEF HISTORY OF SENEGAL

1. Over 95 percent of Senegal's population identifies as Muslim.
2. *Le Sénégal peut-il sortir de la crise?*
3. The four *communes* were Saint Louis, Rufisque, Gorée, and Dakar.
4. Boone emphasizes Cruise O'Brien's remark that by the 1950s politics was the single greatest source of revenue for the Murid elite (Cruise O'Brien 1972, 262 cited in Boone 1992).
5. For a lengthier examination of the failures of the Manatali and Diama dam projects, see Adams 2000.
6. Senghor orchestrated the handing of power to Abdou Diouf by retiring in 1981, which ensured that the prime minister would serve as president until the next election cycle. Although this smooth transition reflects the dominance of the UPS party, there was little economic optimism during Diouf's twenty-year reign as president.
7. Wade was reelected for a second term in 2007, but his presidency has failed to generate much enthusiasm among the Senegalese populace, and even less among the intellectual elite.

CHAPTER 3   URBAN AND RURAL DILEMMAS

1. This designation comes from Wolof, *dëkk bu wow*, which translates literally as dry city, but means a poor city where very little money circulates. This is an ironic label for Saint Louis, as water in many forms, from the Senegal River to annual flooding during the rainy season, has plagued residents since the city's creation.
2. A *bidonville* is an area in which residents have created haphazard dwellings with scrap materials they obtain for free or at very low cost.
3. These titles designate the traditional authorities in Senegal's precolonial kingdoms.
4. Diagne (1919) cites Faidherbe for this estimate. He also documented that half of these revenues went to the local population, while half went to the Damel. Witherell (1964) claims that the annual revenue was in the neighborhood of 50,000FF.
5. Although less common now, historically Wolof marriage patterns demonstrated a preference for marrying cross-cousins. The majority of husbands and wives in Daru-Mumbaay are related in some way, often on both the maternal and paternal sides of each spouse.
6. The remaining five household heads were older men who were once wealthy but are now financially dependent on their children.

CHAPTER 4   GLOBAL HEALTH REFORM IN SAINT LOUIS

1. For a longer discussion of Senegal's reproductive health policies and experiences with family planning programs, see Foley 2007.

2. These include education on common health problems and how to treat and prevent them, promoting good nutrition, access to clean water, promoting maternal and child health, vaccinations, prevention of endemic diseases, providing treatment for common diseases, and maintaining supplies of essential medicines.

3. Monitoring is based on evaluating monthly reports, epidemiological data, and consultation-visit data, all of which the head nurses were withholding as part of the ongoing information boycott.

4. Mr. Seck has been quite vocal in his opposition politics and wanted recognition for his insights; therefore his name has not been changed.

5. He is now a high-ranking official at the Ministry of Health in Dakar.

CHAPTER 5   MARKET-BASED MEDICINE
AND SHANTYTOWN POLITICS IN PIKINE

1. "Ku feebar Pikine, doo fajoo Pikine."

2. "Notre poste de santé est malade."

3. This partnership is based on a "sister city" relationship between Lille, France, and Saint Louis. The annual budget of the Lille office in Saint Louis exceeds several hundred thousand dollars.

4. One of the Health Committee members of the Gut Ndar committee confided to me that they had worked out a similar system with their ICP, who receives a financial bonus every month along with other staff members. He emphasized that this strategy was geared less at motivating the personnel than in keeping them quiet and preventing them from intervening in Health Committee affairs. He suggested that the head nurse would not get in their way as he has a vested interest in receiving his financial bonus every month.

5. "Xëy na tendances politiques yi ñoo bari."

6. I later learned from Seck that some of Joob's problems stemmed from a bitter divorce, one that had humiliated him and in which he was absorbed to the point of being unable to work regularly.

7. In Joob's case it was said that he was treating patients privately out of his home, so indeed he had abandoned his work at the dispensary to work elsewhere. He was purported to be studying law at the University of Saint Louis, and he requested that I send him brochures on MPH programs in the United States. By the end of my field research period, he had enrolled in a computer and technology course. In early 2000 he e-mailed me from New York asking me to send him a copy of the photograph I had taken of him at the Pikine health post.

CHAPTER 6   KNOWLEDGE ENCOUNTERS

1. Although obesity can be an index of household food security, in many cases the urban poor are at risk of becoming obese because their diets consist largely of white rice, bread, macaroni, and oils.

2. "Drinking verses" means writing medicinal verses from the Koran on a piece of paper that is then dissolved in water and ingested, or else writing them on a chalk board, washing the words off the board, and drinking the resulting water.

3. *Yalla yalla bey sa tol.*

CHAPTER 7 GENDER, SOCIAL HIERARCHY, AND HEALTH PRACTICE

1. The onion harvest of 2001 was exceptional and the bride-price rose to 900,000FCFA (US$1,285).

2. Although Senegal's Family Code has provided an alternative to Islamic law that gives women additional rights in circumstances of marriage, divorce, and widowhood, even in this more "progressive" civil law men are the legal heads of household.

3. In the early 1990s an Italian development project equipped most of Ganjool with water taps and small water towers. The water is pumped in from a water treatment plant. Most households are less than 50 yards from a water tap, which has significantly reduced the amount of time women spend obtaining water. Now the most difficult aspect of getting water is working around the erratic schedule of the water tap operators. In Ngeyeen the "water mistress" is a crabby older woman who often inconveniences everyone by delaying the tap's opening in the morning, closing early, and so on.

4. Obtaining the DQ is a constant worry and challenge for rural and urban household heads alike. In the past decade a cartoonist has created a popular character named "Goorgoorlu" (which literally means to struggle in Wolof), most of whose exploits revolve around trying to get the DQ every day to appease his nagging wife.

CHAPTER 8 DOMESTIC DISPUTES AND GENERATIONAL STRUGGLES OVER HOUSEHOLD HEALTH

1. In their research in Guinea, Leach et al. 2008 found that the gendered nature of therapeutic spaces, particularly the "femaleness" of primary health centers, was a key criterion in treatment decisions.

2. Her husband had emigrated to Italy and her frequent pursuit of biomedical treatment could be interpreted as conspicuous consumption enabled by her husband's new-found wealth.

CHAPTER 9 ENCOUNTERING DEVELOPMENT IN GANJOOL

1. Plan International is a large development agency that focuses its work on children and families. It receives most of its funding through child sponsorship. There was a regional Plan International office in Saint Louis, and it was the only NGO working in Ganjool during my field research.

2. See Dettwyler (1993) for a contrasting analysis of the ways that a lack of understanding of the connection between nutrition and child development, and cultural understandings of malnutrition, influence child feeding in Mali.

3. When I was conducting my own household survey, many people asked why I was collecting the information and if I would be bringing a development project. Some people also told me that they were only giving me information because I was

an in-law. I thought this was an exaggeration at the time, but after hearing about the problems with Plan International I realized that they had actually declined to give information to others conducting similar surveys.

CHAPTER 10 BELIEVE IN GOD, BUT PLOW YOUR FIELD

1. As mentioned in chapter 3, by 2008 two of these sons had successfully made it to Europe in an open-air fishing boat.

GLOSSARY
(WOLOF AND FRENCH TERMS)

animation rurale. rural development

attaya. tea

baadoolo. poor

bana-bana. merchant

ber kër. to establish one's own household

bidonville. shantytown

borom kër. owner or head of a household

borom neg. head of the bedroom

boubou. long flowing robe

brak. ruler of Waalo

car-rapide. public transport vehicle

commune. administrative district

comptoir. trading post

damel. ruler of Cajoor

dekk bu wow. poor town

dem. shape-shifters that consume human flesh

doxaan. courting

DQ (dépenses quotidiennes). daily household expenses

drianke. attractive middle-aged woman

entrepôt. trade depot

fajjkat. healer

feebar u Wolof. a Wolof illness

garab u tubaab. European medicine

garab u Wolof. Wolof medicine

halal. acceptable

haram, forbidden

ICP (infirmier-chef de poste). head nurse

jëgg. to transport goods by camel

jinne. evil spirit

jumaa. Friday mosque

kilifa. authority figure

laabiir. compassionate

lambatu. to go back and forth

lotissement. zoning

marabout. Muslim leader or scholar

MD (médecin-chef). head doctor

métis. Creole or mixed-race

mocc. traditional healing technique involving massage and body manipulations

mocckat. healer who practices mocc

mokk pooj. ensuring marital harmony by complying with female gender norms

mool. fisherman

ndëp. healing ceremony for mental illness and spirit possession

postes de santé. health posts

quartier non-loti. unplanned neighborhoods

rabb. ancestral spirits

responsibilization [French]. to make someone take responsibility

sabar. drum

sëriñ. Muslim cleric, also a healer

sharia. Islamic law

sibiiru. malaria

sonsaa. red onions

sutuura. discretion

suurga. stranger or foreigner

suutuura. privacy or discretion

tariqa. Sufi order

tas. chronic tiredness

tension. hypertension

tooy. illness due to overwork and depletion

tubaab. Westerner, usually French

tuul. remedy for protection against metal weapons

tuur. tea drinking party

wujj. co-wife

xiiboon. skinny

REFERENCES

Abu-Lughod, L. 1991. "Writing against Culture." In *Recapturing Anthropology: Working in the Present.* Edited by R. Fox. Santa Fe, N.M.: School of American Research Press.

———. 1993. *Writing Women's Worlds: Bedouin Stories.* Berkeley: University of California Press.

Adams, A. 2000. *The Senegal River: Flood Management and the Future of the Valley.* Washington, D.C.: International Food Policy Research Institute.

Arce, A., and N. Long, eds. 2000. *Anthropology, Development and Modernities: Exploring Discourses, Counter-Tendencies and Violence.* London: Routledge.

Asher, K. 2009. *Black and Green: Afro-Columbians, Development and Nature in the Pacific Lowlands of Colombia.* Durham, N.C.: Duke University Press.

Babou, C. A. M. 1997. "Autour de la Genèse du Mouridisme." *Islam et Sociétés au Sud du Sahara* 11:5–36.

———. 2007. *Fighting the Greater Jihad: Amadu Bamba and the Founding of the Muridiyya of Senegal, 1853–1913.* Athens: Ohio University Press.

Baer, H. A. 1996. "Bringing Political Ecology into Critical Medical Anthropology: A Challenge to Biocultural Approaches." *Medical Anthropology* 17:129–141.

———. 1997. "The Misconception of Critical Medical Anthropology: A Response to a Cultural Constructivist Critique." *Social Science and Medicine* 44(10):1565–1573.

Baer, H., M. Singer, and I. Susser. 2004. *Medical Anthropology and the World System.* Westport, Conn.: Praeger.

Baer, H. A., M. Singer, and J. Johnsen. 1986. "Toward a Critical Medical Anthropology." *Social Science and Medicine* 23(2):95–98.

Barry, B. 1972. *Le Royaume du Walo, 1659–1859: Le Sénégal Avant la Conquête.* Paris: Maspero.

———. 1985. *Le royaume du Waalo: Le Sénégal avant la conqête.* Paris: Karthala.

———. 1997. *Senegambia and the Atlantic Slave Trade.* Cambridge: Cambridge University Press.

Beckerleg, S. 1994. "Medical Pluralism and Islam in Swahili Communities in Kenya." *Medical Anthropology Quarterly* 8(3):199–213.

Blas, E., and N. Hearst. 2002. "Health Sector Reform and Equity—Learning from Evidence?" *Health Policy and Planning* 17(Suppl. 1):1–4.

Bloom, G., and H. Standing. 2008. "Future Health Systems: Why Future? Why Now?" *Social Science and Medicine* 66(10):2067–2075.

Bloom, G., H. Standing, and R. Lloyd. 2008. "Markets, Information Asymmetry, and Health Care: Towards New Social Contracts." *Social Science and Medicine* 66(10):2076–2087.

Bonnardel, R. 1992. *Saint Louis du Sénégal: Mort ou Naissance?* Paris: Harmattan.

Boone, C. 1992. *Merchant Capital and the Roots of State Power in Senegal, 1930–1985.* Cambridge: Cambridge University Press.

———. 2003. *Political Topographies of the African State: Territorial Authority and Institutional Choice.* Cambridge: Cambridge University Press.

Boulegue, J. 1987. *Le Grand Jolof.* Paris: Editions Karthala.

Bourdieu, P. 1977. *Outline of a Theory of Practice.* Cambridge: Cambridge University Press.

Boye, M. Y. 1984. "Rapport introductive sur les problèmes d'urbanisme et d'habitat de la ville de Saint-Louis." Saint Louis: Commission Régional de l'Urbanisme, Ministère de l'Urbanisme et de l'Habitat, République du Sénégal.

Brodwin, P. 1996. *Medicine and Morality in Haiti: The Contest for Healing Power.* Cambridge: Cambridge University Press.

Buggenhagen, B. 2004. "Domestic Object(ion)s: The Senegalese Murid Trade Diaspora and the Politics of Marriage Payments, Love, and State Privatization." In *Producing African Futures: Ritual and Reproduction in a Neoliberal Age.* Edited by B. Weiss, 21–53. Leiden: Brill Academic Press.

Camera, C. 1968. *Saint Louis du Sénégal: Évolution d'une ville en Milieu Africain.* Dakar: IFAN.

Carillo, H. 2002. *The Night Is Young: Sexuality in Mexico in a Time of AIDS.* Chicago: University of Chicago Press.

Castro, A., and M. Singer. 2004. Introduction to *Unhealthy Health Policy.* Edited by A. Castro and M. Singer, 11–20. Lanham, Md.: AltaMira Press.

Collins C., and A. Green. 1994. "Decentralization and Primary Health Care: Some Negative Implications in Developing Countries." *International Journal of Health Services* 24:461.

Cornia, G. A. 1987. "Adjustment at the Household Level: Potential and Limitations of Survival Strategies." In *Adjustment with a Human Face.* Edited by G. A. Cornia, R. Jolly, and F. Stewart. Vol. 1. Oxford: Clarendon Press.

Cornwall, A., and A. Shankland. 2008. "Engaging Citizens: Lessons from Building Brazil's National Health System." *Social Science and Medicine* 66(10):2173–2184.

Coulibaly, A. L. 2003. *Wade, un opposant au pouvoir: L'alternance Piégée?* Dakar: Les Editions Sentinelles.

Crandon-Malamud, L. 1991. *From the Fat of Our Souls: Social Change, Political Process, and Medical Pluralism in Bolivia.* Berkeley: University of California Press.

Creese, A. L. 1990. *User Charges for Health Care: A Review of Recent Experience.* Geneva: World Health Organization.

Crowder, M. 1967. *Senegal: A Study of French Assimilation Policy.* London: Metheun.

———. 1968. *West Africa under Colonial Rule.* Evanston, Ill.: Northwestern University Press.

Csordas, T., and A. Kleinman. 1990. "The Therapeutic Process." In *Medical Anthropology: Contemporary Theory and Method.* Edited by T. Johnson and C. Sargent, 11–25. New York: Praeger.

Curtin, P. 1972. *The Atlantic Slave Trade: A Census.* Madison: University of Wisconsin Press.

Derman, W., F. Gonesse, and C. Chikozho. 2000. "Decentralization, Devolution, and Development: Reflections on the Water Reform Process in Zimbabwe." Paper presented at the BASIS CRSP Workshop on Water, University of Malawi.

Dettwyler, K. 1993. *Dancing Skeletons: Life and Death in West Africa.* Long Grove, Ill.: Waveland Press.

Dia, A. 1999. *Impacts des aménagements hydrauliques du Fleuve Sénégal sur les écosystèmes humides du delta.* Dakar: Union Mondiale pour la Nature.

Dia, P. I. 1998. "Gestion urbaine et pratiques sociales dans les villes du Tiers-Monde: L'exemple de Pikine à Saint Louis du Sénégal." Mémoire de DEA, Institut d'Urbanisme de Grenoble.

Diagne, A. M. 1919. "Un Pays de Pilleurs d'Épaves: Le Gandiole." *Bulletin du Comité d'Études Historique et Scientifiques de l'AOF,* 1 January, 137–176.

Diop, A. B. 1981. *La société Wolof.* Paris: Karthala.

———. 1985. *La famille Wolof: Tradition et changement.* Paris: Karthala.

Diop, M. C. 2002. *La société Sénégalaise entre le local et le global.* Paris: Editions Karthala.

———. 2004. *Gouverner le Sénégal: Entre ajustement structurel et développement durable.* Paris: Editions Karthala.

Diouf, M. 1990. *Le Kajoor au XIXe siècle: Pouvoir Ceddo et conquête coloniale.* Paris: Éditions Karthala.

———. 1998. "The French Colonial Policy of Assimilation and the Civility of the Originaires of the Four Communes (Senegal): A Nineteenth Century Globalization Project." *Development and Change* 29:671–696.

———. 2001. *Histoire du Sénégal: Le modèle Islamo-Wolof et ses périphéries.* Paris: Maisonneuve et Larose.

Doyal, L. 1979. *The Political Economy of Health.* London: Pluto Press.

Duruflé, G. 1994. *Le Sénégal peut-il sortir de la crise? Douze ans d'ajustement structurel au Sénégal.* Paris: Karthala.

Engelberg, G. 2005. "Question Success: Did Senegal Do the Right Thing, Or Is the Worst of AIDS Yet to Come?" *World View Magazine* Vol. 18, no. 2 (September).

Evans, T., M. Whitehead, F. Diderichsen, A. Bhuiya, and M. Wirth, eds. 2001. *Challenging Inequities in Health: From Ethics to Action.* Oxford: Oxford University Press.

Evans-Pritchard, E. E. 1937. *Witchcraft, Oracles, and Magic among the Azande.* London: Clarendon Press.

Farmer, P. 1993. *AIDS and Accusation.* Berkeley: University of California Press.

———. 1997. "On Suffering and Structural Violence: A View from Below." In *Social Suffering.* Edited by A. Kleinman, V. Das, and M. Lock. Berkeley: University of California Press.

———. 2001. *Infections and Inequalities: The Modern Plagues.* Berkeley: University of California Press.

———. 2004. "An Anthropology of Structural Violence." *Current Anthropology* 45(3): 305–317.

———. 2005. *Pathologies of Power: Health, Human Rights, and the New War on the Poor.* Berkeley: University of California Press.

Fassin, D. 1992. *Pouvoir et maladie en Afrique: Anthropologie sociale dans la banlieue de Dakar.* Paris: Presses Universitaires de France.

Fassin, E., and D. Fassin. 1988. "De la quête de légitimation à la question de la légitimité: Les thérapeutiques "traditionnelles" au Sénégal." *Cahier d'Études Africaines* 110(XXVIII-2):207–231.

Feierman, S. 1985. "Struggles for Control: The Social Roots of Health and Healing in Modern Africa." *African Studies Review* 28(2, 3):73–147.

Feierman, S., and J. Janzen, eds. 1992. *The Social Basis of Health and Healing in Africa.* Berkeley: University of California Press.

Ferguson, J. 1994. *The Anti-politics Machine: "Development," Depoliticization, and Bureaucratic Power in Lesotho.* Minneapolis: University of Minnesota Press.

———. 2006. *Global Shadows: Africa in the Neoliberal World Order.* Durham, N.C.: Duke University Press.

Ferguson, J., and A. Gupta. 2002. "Spatializing States: Toward an Ethnography of Neoliberal Governmentality." *American Ethnologist* 29(4):981–1002.

Foley, E. 2001. "No Money, No Care: Women and Health Sector Reform in Senegal." *Urban Anthropology and Studies of Cultural Systems and World Economic Development* 30(1):1–50.

———. 2007. "Overlaps and Disconnects in Reproductive Health Care: Global Policies, National Programs, and the Micropolitics of Fertility and Contraceptive Use in Northern Senegal." *Medical Anthropology* 26(4):323–354.

————. 2008. "Neoliberal Reform and Health Dilemmas: Illness, Social Hierarchy, and Therapeutic Decision-Making in Senegal." *Medical Anthropology Quarterly* 22(3): 257–273.

Foote, K. A., K. H. Hill, and L. G. Martin, eds. 1993. *Demographic Change in Sub-Saharan Africa*. Washington, D.C.: National Academies Press.

Fort, M., M. A. Mercer, and O. Gish, eds. 2004. *Sickness and Wealth: The Corporate Assault on Global Health*. Cambridge, Mass.: South End Press.

Frank, G. 1969. "The Development of Underdevelopment." *Monthly Review* 18(4).

Frankenberg, R. 1974. "Functionalism and After? Theory and Developments in Social Science Applied to the Health Field." *International Journal of Health Services* 4(3):411–427.

Gaines, A. 1991. "Cultural Constructivism: Sickness Histories and the Understanding of Ethnomedicines beyond Critical Medical Anthropologies." In *Anthropologies of Medicine: A Colloquium on Western European and American Perspectives*. Edited by G. Bibeau. Wiesbeden, Germany: Verlag Vieweg.

Galvan, D. 2004. *The State Must Be Our Master of Fire: How Peasants Craft Culturally Sustainable Development*. Berkeley: University of California Press.

Gamble, D. 1957. *The Wolof of Senegambia*. London: International African Institute.

Gellar, S. 1982. *Senegal: An African Nation between Islam and the West*. Boulder, Colo.: Westview Press.

————. 2005. *Democracy in Senegal: Tocquevillian Analytics in Africa*. New York: Palgrave Macmillan.

Gwatkin, D. R. 2001. "The Need for Equity-Oriented Health Sector Reforms." *International Journal of Epidemiology* 30:720–723.

Harding, S. 1991. *Whose Science? Whose Knowledge?* Ithaca, N.Y.: Cornell University Press.

Harney, E. 2004. *In Senghor's Shadow: Art, Politics, and the Avante-Garde in Senegal, 1960–1995*. Durham, N.C.: Duke University Press.

Hong, E. 2004. "The Primary Health Care Movement Meets the Free Market." In *Sickness and Wealth: The Corporate Assault on Global Health*. Edited by M. Fort, M. A. Mercer, and O. Gish, 27–36. Cambridge, Mass.: South End Press.

Horton, R. 1967. "African Traditional Thought and Western Science." *Africa* 37 (1 & 2).

Houma, Y. 1991. "Etude Démographique d'un Quartier Périphérique de Saint Louis: Goxumbacc." Master's thesis, Université Cheikh Anta Diop.

Janes, C. 2003. "Market Fetishism and Attenuated Primary Care: Producing Poor Medicine for Poor People in Post-Socialist Mongolia." *Bulletin of the Royal Institute for Interfaith Studies* 5(1):43–68.

————. 2004. "Going Global in Century Twenty-One: Medical Anthropology and the New Primary Health Care." *Human Organization* 63(4):457–471.

Janes, C., and O. Chuluundorj. 2004. "Free Markets and Dead Mothers: The Social Ecology of Maternal Mortality in Post-Socialist Mongolia." *Medical Anthropology Quarterly* 18(2):102–129.

Janes, C. R., et al. 2006. "Poor Medicine for Poor People? Assessing the Impact of Neoliberal Reform on Health Care Equity in a Post-Socialist Context." *Global Public Health* 1(1):5–30.

Janzen, J. 1978. *The Quest for Therapy: Medical Pluralism in Lower Zaire*. Berkeley: University of California Press.

Johnson, W. 1971. *The Emergence of Black Politics in Senegal, 1900–1920*. Palo Alto, Calif.: Stanford University Press.

Jurgens, R. and F.L. Dia. 2006. *Leadership in Action: A Case Study of the "Observatoire," a Group of NGOs in Senegal*. Dakar: International HIV/AIDS Alliance.

Kanji, N. 1989. "Charging for Drugs in Africa: UNICEF's Bamako Initiative." *Health Policy and Planning* 4(2):110–120.

Keita, M. 1996. "The Political Economy of Health Care in Senegal." *Journal of Asian and African Studies* 31(3, 4):145–161.

———. 2006. *A Political Economy of Health Care in Senegal*. Leiden: Brill.

Kim, J. Y., et al., eds. 2000. *Dying for Growth: Global Inequality and the Health of the Poor*. Monroe, Maine: Common Courage Press.

Kleinman, A. 1980. *Patients and Healers in the Context of Culture*. Berkeley: University of California Press.

———. 1986. "Social Origins of Distress and Disease." *Current Anthropology* 27(5):499–509.

———. 1992. "Pain and Resistance: The Delegitimation and Relegitimation of Local Worlds." In *Pain as Human Experience: An Anthropological Perspective*. Edited by M. J. D. Good et al., 169–197. Berkeley: University of California Press.

Lambek, M. 1993. *Knowledge and Practice in Mayotte: Local Discourses of Islam, Sorcery, and Spirit Possession*. Toronto: University of Toronto Press.

Last, M. 1992. "The Importance of Knowing about Not Knowing: Observations from Hausaland." In *The Social Basis of Health and Healing in Africa*. Edited by S. Feierman and J. Janzen, 393–408. Berkeley: University of California Press.

Leach, M. A., et al. 2008. "New Therapeutic Landscapes in Africa: Parental Categories and Practices in Seeking Infant Health in the Republic of Guinea." *Social Science and Medicine* 66:2157–2167.

Leonard, K. 2007. "Learning in Health Care: Evidence of Learning about Clinician Quality in Tanzania." *Economic Development and Cultural Change* 55(3):533–555.

Leslie, C., ed. 1976. *Asian Medical Systems: A Comparative Study*. Berkeley: University of California Press.

Leys, C. 1996. *The Rise and Fall of Development Theory*. Bloomington: Indiana University Press.

Lo, M. G., O. Ndiaye, and M. Toure. 1997. *Étude relative à la problématique des comités de santé dans le développement sanitaire*. Dakar: Cabinet International de Conseil et d'Étude pour le Développement.

Lock, M., and N. Scheper-Hughes. 1990. "A Critical-Interpretive Approach in Medical Anthropology: Rituals and Routines of Discipline and Dissent." In *Medical Anthropology: Contemporary Theory and Method*. Edited by T. Johnson and C. Sargent, 47–72. New York: Praeger.

———. 1987. "The Mindful Body: A Prolegomenon to Future Work in Medical Anthropology." *Medical Anthropology Quarterly* 1:6–41.

Long, N., and A. Long, eds. 1992. *Battlefields of Knowledge: The Interlocking of Theory and Practice in Social Research and Development*. London: Routledge.

Luedke, T., and H. West, eds. 2006. *Borders and Healers: Brokering Therapeutic Resources in Southeast Africa*. Bloomington: Indiana University Press.

Ly, I. 1997. "Exploitation des données du recensement de Pikine Saint Louis du 26 Août au 8 Septembre 1996." Saint Louis: Cellule Base de Données Urbaines de la D.U.A., Direction de l'Urbanisme et de l'Architecture.

Marcus, G. 1995. "Ethnography in/of the World System: The Emergence of Multi-Sited Ethnography." *Annual Review of Anthropology* 24:95–117.

Marcus, G., and M. Fischer. 1986. *Anthropology as Cultural Critique*. Chicago: University of Chicago Press.

McMichael, P. 1996. "Globalization: Myths and Realities." *Rural Sociology* 61:1–20.

Meinert, L. 2004. "Resources for Health in Uganda: Bourdieu's Concepts of Capital and Habitus." *Anthropology and Medicine* 11(1):11–26.

Ministère de l'Economie, des Finances et du Plan. 1998. "Évaluation du processus de planification dans le contexte de la régionalisation: Rapport d'une étude dans les régions de Fatick, Kaolack, Louga et Saint Louis." Dakar: République du Sénégal.

Ministére de la Sante Publique et de la Prévention Médicale. 2005. *Enquête Démographique et de Santé (EDS-IV)*. Dakar: Sénégal.

———. 2006. *Sénégal enquête démographique et de Santé, rapport préliminaire*. Dakar, Sénégal: Centre de Recherche pour le Développement Humain. Calverton, Maryland: MEASURE DHS+, ORC Macro.

———. 2006. *Annuaire statistique 2005, version finale*. Dakar, Sénégal: Service Nationale de l'Information Sanitaire.

Morgan, L. 1987. "Dependency Theory in the Political Economy of Health: An Anthropological Critique." *Medical Anthropology Quarterly* 1(2):131–155.

Morsy, S. 1979. "The Missing Link in Medical Anthropology: The Political Economy of Health." *Reviews in Anthropology* 6:349–363.

———. 1981. "Towards a Political Economy of Health: A Critical Note on the Medical Anthropology of the Middle East." *Social Science and Medicine* 15(b):159–163.

———. 1990. "Political Economy in Medical Anthropology." In *Medical Anthropology: Contemporary Theory and Method*. Edited by T. Johnson and C. Sargent, 26–46. New York: Praeger.

Ndiaye, A. 1987. "Étude d'une extension périphérique: Pikine." B.A., University Cheikh Anta Diop.

Ndiaye S., M. Ayad, and A. Gaye. 1997. *Enquête démographique et de santé au Sénégal (EDS-III)*. Dakar, Sénégal: Ministère de l'Économie, des Finances et du Plan, Direction de la Prévision et de la Statistique, Division des Statistiques Démographiques; Calverton, Md.: Macro International.

Ndiaye S., P. D. Diouf, and M. Ayad. 1992/93. *Enquête démographique et de santé au Sénégal (EDS-II)*. Dakar: Ministère de l'Économie, des Finances, et du Plan, Direction de la Prévision et de la Statistique, Division des Statistiques Démographiques.

Ndiaye S., I. Saar, and M. Ayad. 1986. *Enquête démographique et de santé au Sénégal (EDS-I)*. Dakar, Sénégal: Ministère de l'Économie, des Finances et du Plan, Direction de la Prévision et de la Statistique, Division des Statistiques Démographiques; Calverton, Md.: Macro International.

Ngalamulume, K. 1996. "City Growth, Health Problems, and Colonial Government Response: Saint Louis (Senegal) from the Mid-Nineteenth Century to the First World War." Ph.D. Dissertation, Michigan State University.

Nguyen, V. K., and K. Peschard. 2003. "Anthropology, Inequality, and Disease: A Review." *Annual Review of Anthropology* 32:447–474.

Nyamnjoh, F. 2005. "Fishing in Troubled Waters: Disquettes and Thiofs in Dakar." *Africa* 75(3):295–324.

Obbo, C. 1996. "Healing Cultural Fundamentalism and Cultural Syncreticism in Buganda, Africa." *Journal of the International African Institute* 66(2):183–201.

Obrist, B. 2003. "Urban Health in Daily Practice: Livelihood, Vulnerability, and Resilience in Dar es Salaam, Tanzania." *Anthropology and Medicine* 10(3):275–290.

Ortner, S. 1984. "Theory in Anthropology since the Sixties." *Comparative Studies in Society and History* 26(1):126–166.

———. 2006. *Anthropology and Social Theory: Culture, Power, and the Acting Subject*. Durham, N.C.: Duke University Press.

Paluzzi, J. 2004. "Primary Health Care since Alma Ata: Lost in the Bretton Woods?" In *Unhealthy Health Policy*. Edited by A. Castro and M. Singer, 63–77. Lanham, Md.: AltaMira Press.

Peters, P. E., ed. 2000. *Development Encounters: Sites of Participation and Knowledge*. Cambridge, Mass.: Harvard University Press.

Peter, F., and Evans, T. 2001. "Ethical Dimensions of Health Equity: Challenging Inequities". In *Health: From Ethics to Action*. Edited by T. Evans et al., 25–33. Oxford: Oxford University Press.

Pfeiffer, J., and M. Nichter. 2008. "What Can Critical Medical Anthropology Contribute to Global Health?" *Medical Anthropology Quarterly* 22(4):410–415.

Pigg, S. L. 2005. "Globalizing the Facts of Life." In *Sex in Development: Science, Sexuality, and Morality in Global Perspective*. Edited by V. Adams and S. Pigg, 39–69. Durham, N.C.: Duke University Press.

Population Reference Bureau. 2007. *World Population Data Sheet*. Washington, D.C.: Population Reference Bureau.

———. 2008. *World Population Data Sheet*. Washington, D.C.: Population Reference Bureau.

Ridde, V. 2003. "Entre efficacité et qualité: Qu'en est-il de l'initiative de Bamako? Une revue des expériences Ouest-Africaines." Paper presented at the 26th Journées des Economistes Français de la Santé, Santé et Développement, Clermont-Ferrand.

Roberts, M. J., and M. R. Reich. 2002. "Ethical Analysis in Public Health." *The Lancet* 359:1055–1059.

Roberts, M. J., W. Hsiao, P. Berman, and M. R. Reich. 2004. *Getting Health Reform Right*. Oxford: Oxford University Press.

Robinson, D. 2000. *Paths of Accommodation: Muslim Societies and French Colonial Authorities in Senegal and Mauritania, 1880–1920*. Athens: Ohio University Press.

Robinson, D., and J.-L. Triaud, eds. 1997. *Le temps des marabouts: Itinéraires et stratégies islamiques en Afrique Occidentale Française, v.1880–1960*. Paris: Editions Karthala.

Rodney, W. 1973. *How Europe Underdeveloped Africa*. London: Bogle-L'Overture Publications.

Rosaldo, R. 1993. *Culture and Truth: The Remaking of Social Analysis*. Boston: Beacon Press.

Scheper-Hughes, N. 1993. *Death without Weeping: The Violence of Everyday Life in Brazil*. Berkeley: University of California Press.

Schoepf, B., C. Schoepf, and J. Millen. 2000. "Theoretical Therapies, Remote Remedies: SAPS and the Political Ecology of Poverty and Health in Africa." In *Dying for Growth: Global Inequality and the Health of the Poor*. Edited by J. Y. Kim et al. Monroe, Maine: Common Courage Press.

Shaw, P., and C. Griffin. 1995. *Financing Health Care in Sub-Saharan Africa through User Fees and Insurance*. Washington, D.C.: World Bank.

Singer, M. 1986. "Developing a Critical Perspective in Medical Anthropology." *Medical Anthropology Quarterly* 17(5):128–129.

———. 1989. "The Coming of Age of Critical Medical Anthropology." *Social Science and Medicine* 28(11):1193–1203.

———. 1990. "Reinventing Medical Anthropology: Toward a Critical Realignment." *Social Science and Medicine* 30(2):179–187.

Smith, R., and P. Siplon. 2006. *Drugs into Bodies: Global AIDS Treatment Activism*. Westport, Conn.: Praeger.

Sparr, Pamela, ed. 1994. *Mortgaging Women's Lives*. London: Zed Books.

Spierenberg, M., D. Diop, and M. Eza. 1999. *Rapport de mission: Enquête sur la décentralisation au Sénégal*. Dakar: Projet UNESCO, DANIDA, IAD.

Thomas-Emeagwali, G. 1995. "Introductory Perspectives: Monetarists, Liberals and Radicals: Contrasting Perspectives on Gender and Structural Adjustment." In *Women Pay the Price: Structural Adjustment in Africa and the Caribbean*. Edited by G. Thomas-Emeagwali. Trenton, N.J.: Africa World Press.

Turner, V. 1967. *The Forest of Symbols*. Ithaca, N.Y.: Cornell University Press.

Turshen, M. 1984. *The Political Ecology of Disease in Tanzania*. New Brunswick, N.J.: Rutgers University Press.

———. 1999. *Privatizing Health Services in Africa*. New Brunswick, N.J.: Rutgers University Press.

UICN/Réseau National Zones Humides. 1999. "Élaboration d'un plan de gestion intégrée des zones humides de la périphérie de Saint-Louis et du Gandiolais. Dakar: UICN.

UNICEF. 1987. *Adjustment with a Human Face: Protecting the Vulnerable and Promoting Growth*. New York: UNICEF.

UNICEF-WHO. 1991. "The Bamako Initiative Progress Report: A UNICEF Assessment. UNICEF-WHO Joint Committee on Health Policy document JCKP28/91/18." Geneva: UNICEF-WHO.

United Nations. 1989. *Demographic Yearbook, 1987*. New York: United Nations.

Vaughan, M. 1991. *Curing Their Ills: Colonial Power and African Illness*. Cambridge, U.K.: Polity Press.

Villalon, L. 1995. *Islamic Society and State Power in Senegal*. Cambridge: Cambridge University Press.

Wallerstein, I. 1979. *The Capitalist World-Economy*. London: Cambridge University Press.

Webster, Neil. 1992. "Panchayati Raj in West Bengal: Popular Participation for the People or the Party?" *Development and Change* 23(4):129–163.

Weston, K. 1991. *Families We Choose: Lesbians, Gays, Kinship*. New York: Columbia University Press.

Whiteford, L., and L. Manderson, eds. 2000. *Global Health Policy, Local Realities: The Myth of the Level Playing Field*. Boulder, Colo.: Lynne Rienner Publishers.

Witherell, J. 1964. "The Response of the Peoples of Cayor to French Penetration, 1850–1900." Ph.D. Dissertation, University of Wisconsin.

World Bank. 1987. "Financing Health Services in Developing Countries: An Agenda for Reform." Washington, D.C.: World Bank.

———. 1993. "World Development Report: Investing in Health." Washington, D.C.: World Bank.

———. World Development Indicators. http://web.worldbank.org/WBSITE/EXTERNAL/DATASTATISTICS/0,,contentMDK:21725423~pagePK:64133150~piPK:64133175~theSitePK:239419,00.html (accessed on January 16, 2009).

Zemplini, A. 1968. "L'interprétation et la thérapie traditionnelle du désordre mental chez les Wolof et les Lébou du Sénégal." Thèse de 3e Cycle en Ethnologie, Paris.

INDEX

Italicized page numbers refer to figures and tables.

Abu-Lughod, Lila, 7–8
accountability, 5, 68, 70, 82, 95
activism, 3, 62–63, 68
administrators, 4–5, 11–12, 27–28;
    epidemiological data from, 64; and global
    health reform, 58–59, 69–72, 76, 160; and
    Pikine health post, 88, 94
African socialism, 20, 28–29, 31–32, 36
Afrique Occidental Française (AOF), 25–28,
    37, 40
agriculture, 25–26, 30–31, 164; in Ganjool,
    17, 38, 40, 46, 52–55, 119, 144, 154; history
    of, 47–50, 56–57; and politics of gender
    and household, 119–121, 125. *See also*
    onion farming; peanut production/trade
AIDS. *See* HIV/AIDS
Alma Ata Conference (1978), 5, 17, 59
amulets, 100, 110, 113, 125
anemia, 105, 107, 127
animation rurale (rural development), 31
Annuaire Statistique (2005), 64
anthropology, 4, 7–11, 14–17, 99, 155,
    158–159
antiretroviral medication, 68
aspirin, 87, 103
assimilation, 26–28, 36
Assistance Médicale Indigène, 24
attaya (tea). *See* tea drinking
austerity programs, 20, 32, 61, 70
authority figure (kilifa), 118, 122–123, 128,
    138–142

baadoolo (poor), 105–106. *See also* poverty
Bamako Initiative, 35, 59–61, 78–82, 85, 91,
    95–96, 128, 160–161
Bamba, Amadu, 22, 27
bana-bana, 48, 51. *See also* traveling
    merchants
bankruptcy, 4, 75, 81, 87–88, 91–95
baptisms, 13, 46, 105, 107, 115, 123
bed nets, 103
begging, 106
bidonvilles. *See* shantytowns
biodiversity, 40, 115
biomedicine, 6, 9, 18, 24, 162–163; and
    development in Ganjool, 146–147, 149,
    156; and family decisions about serious
    illnesses, 133, 135–136, 138, 142, 167n2;

and global health reform, 78–81, 83, 161;
    and health strategies of residents, 96–99,
    101–111, 113; and mothers' concerns for
    child health, 125–126
birth attendants, 65, 68, 103, 149, 153–154,
    156
blood pressure, 97–98
blood screening, 67
borom kër, 118, 122–123, 128, 130, 132,
    141, 146. *See also* household heads
borom neg (head of bedroom), 121–123
Bourdieu, Pierre, 7, 10
brak (ruler of Waalo), 46, 165n3
Brazzaville conference (1944), 28
breast cancer screenings, 6
breastfeeding, 105
brideprice, 49, 117, 167n1

Cajoor, 46, 48, 165nn3,4
camels, 46–48
Canary Islands, 35, 56
cancer, 65, 116, 133, 135
capitalism, 3, 9, 26, 33–35, 37, 62, 160
car-rapides (public transport vehicles), 89
Casamance civil war, 42
case de santé. *See* health huts/health hut
    workers
castes, 20–22
Catholics, 24, 67–68, 109
causerie. *See* health talk
Césaire, Aimé, 28
childbirth, 66–67, *66*, 79, 104, 118, 152–154,
    156, 164
child care, 50, 53, 105, 118, 127–128, 130,
    142
child health, 3, 65, 69, 116, 161, 166n2; and
    development in Ganjool, 145–149, 156,
    167n2; and health strategies of residents,
    99, 103–105, 110; mothers' concerns for,
    124–129
child-sponsorship programs, 6, 15, 149–152,
    167n1
chloroquine, 87, 103, 129, 139
cholera, 65
Christianity, 97
civilizing mission (1854–1960), 25–29
civil society, 26, 61, 68, 77, 82, 94, 161
closed health systems, 99–100

communauté rurale (rural government authority), 145

communes (administrative districts), 26–28, 81, 165n3. *See also* Dakar; Gorée; Rufisque; Saint Louis

community health workers, 13, 68–69, 103, 117

community management. *See* participatory management

Compagnie du Cap Vert, 22–23

competition among healers, 100

condoms, 6, 146–147. *See also* contraception

consultation fees/tickets: and development in Ganjool, 153–154; and global health reform, 68–69, 78–79, 81; and health strategies of residents, 106–107; and mothers' concerns for child health, 128; at Pikine health post, 91–92. *See also* user fees

contraception, 6, 66–67, 107, 146–147

contraception prevalence rate (CPR), 66, *66*

corruption, 73, 82, 85–88, 90–91, 94, 161

cost recovery schemes, 5, 35, 85, 91–92, 95, 103–104, 159, 161. *See also* drug sales; user fees

courtship (doxaan), 117, 119, 121–122, 127

co-wives, 51, 116–118, 120–128, 154–155

credit, 2, 47–48, 50, 105–107, 119, 126, 164

credit agencies, 47, 106, 164

critical medical anthropology (CMA), 5, 9–11, 19; and global health reform, 58–59, 62–63; methods, 11–14; research setting, 4–7

cross-cousin marriages, 165n5

cultural Other, 7–8, 16

currency devaluation (1994), 58

daily household expenses. *See* DQ *(dépenses quotidiennes)*

Dakar, 15, 17, 24–26, 37, 40, 42, 58, 99, 117, 136, 165n3

damel (ruler of Cajoor), 46, 165nn3,4

Daru-Mumbaay, 1–2, 5, 9, 12–16, 19, 115, 164; development in, 144–155; family decisions about serious illnesses in, 130–142; health strategies of residents in, 102–109; history of, 46–51, 57, 165n5; mothers' concerns for child health in, 124–129; politics of gender and household in, 116–124; and sonsaa (red onion) season, 52–55, 115

deaths, 3, 9, 18, 24, 164; from illegal migration, 35, 56; infant/child, 3, 65–67, *66*, 105, 107, 128–129; from malaria, 45, 102; maternal, 3, 65, *66*; PA system used to announce, 47, 103; from poverty, 105; after serious illnesses, 135–136, 164

debts, personal, 2, 48–50, 56, 78, 105–106, 126–127, 138, 157, 164

debts, public: debt crisis, 31, 60–61; at Pikine health post, 86–88, 93

decentralization, 4–5; and global health reform, 17, 58–59, 61, 69–72, 74, 76, 78, 80–83, 160–161; history of in Senegal, 20, 28, 33–34, 37; and Pikine health post, 85, 91, 93–94

De Gaulle, Charles, 28–29

dëkk bu wow (poor town), 40–45, 165n1

dëm (shape-shifters that consume human flesh), 110

democracy, 29–35, 61, 70, 72, 82, 94

Demographic Health Survey (1992), 67

development, 11, 159, 163–164, 167n3; failures of, 6–7, 154–157, 164; in Ganjool, 19, 38, 45–55, 143–157, 167n1; and global health reform, 3–7, 61, 64–65, 72, 161; history of, 28, 31, 33–35, 37–38, 41, 44–55, 57; in Pikine, 86, 91

Dia, Mamadou, 30

diabetes, 65, 79

Diagne, Blaise, 26–27

Diama dam, 17, 31, 37–38, 40, 48, 149, 165n5

diarrheal diseases, 3, 45, 65, 68, 90, 105, 107, 127–128, 162

Diouf, Abdou, 30–32, 165n6

Diouf, Mamadou, 28, 46

diseases, 3, 6, 17, 19, 24, 45; epidemiological data for, 65–67; germ theory of, 24; and global health reform, 59, 61, 82, 166n2; and health strategies of residents, 97–98, 100, 102; power to legitimate, 100. *See also names of diseases*

dispensaries, 4, 12, 88; and global health reform, 60, 68–72, 78–79, 81–82; and health strategies of residents, 103–104, 107–108, 112, 128; history of, 24, 43–44; in Pikine, 84–92, 95. *See also* health clinics; health posts

district staff meetings, 12, 64, 70–71, 74–76, 85, 90–91

district supervisors, 69, 74–76, 94

district training sessions, 12, 69, 75–77, 81–82

diviners, 98, 102

divorce, 123, 166n6, 167n2

doctors, 4–5, 24, 157, 163; and development in Ganjool, 145; and family decisions about serious illnesses, 136, 139; and global health reform, 58, 69, 79–80, 82; and health strategies of residents, 102, 107–108, 112–113. *See also* MC (médecin-chef de district)

donor funding, 6, 65, 68, 81, 86, 89, 91, 94–95, 166n3. *See also* Plan International

doxaan. *See* courtship

DQ *(dépenses quotidiennes)*, 49–51, 116, 118–121, 123, 127, 146, 167n4

drianke (attractive middle-aged woman), 98, 163

"drinking verses," 110, 167n2

droughts, 30, 38, 40, 42–43, 46, 48

drug sales, 2, 5; and global health reform, 60–61, 68–70, 78–81, 161; and health strategies of residents, 106–107; at Pikine dispensary, 85, 87–88, 90–92

"dry city," 40–45, 165n1

dysentery, 15, 127

Economic and Social Development Fund, 28
economic crises, 9, 30, 32
economic policies, 2–5, 8–10, 17–19; and global health reform, 58–60; history of, 20–21, 25–26, 28, 30–35, 37–38, 40–42, 165n6
economic-recovery loans, 31–32
ecotourism, 40, 132
education, 2, 6, 42–44, 48; about HIV/AIDS, 6, 67–68, 146–147, 155; in French colonial era, 20, 23, 26–28; health education, 18, 69, 102, 106, 113, 142, 145, 161, 166n2; higher education, 42, 93, 132–135, 139, 166n7
egalitarian liberal framework, 62–63
elections, 12, 26, 34–35, 73–74, 77, 82, 86, 94, 165nn6,7
electricity, 38, 43–45, 70–72
embezzlement, 85, 88, 90
employment, 2, 38, 41–42, 44–45, 48–52, 55–56, 106, 118–120
endemic diseases, 65, 102, 166n2
endogamous marriages, 22
entrepôt (trade depot), 46
epidemics, 24, 65, 97–98
epidemiological profile, 63–68, 66
eroticism, 122–123, 147–148
essentialism, 8
ethical dilemmas, 61–63
ethnography, 3–4, 10–11, 16, 18–19, 99–101, 159
Europe/Europeans, 15, 22, 24, 40–42

Faidherbe, Louis, 23, 25–26, 165n4
fajjkat (healer in Wolof), 109
families. See households
Family Codes (1972), 35, 167n2
family names, 22, 47
family planning, 6, 65, 69, 107, 109, 162, 166n1
Farmer, Paul, 63
farming. See agriculture
feebar u Wolof (Wolof illness), 133
fees for service. See user fees
Feierman, S., 99–101
feminism, 7, 14
Festival Mondial des Arts Nègres, 32
field research, 11, 16–17
financial management of hospitals/clinics, 2, 4, 69–77, 85–88, 90–95, 103, 166n4. See also drug sales; user fees
Financing Health Services in Developing Countries (World Bank), 60
first-aid procedures, 68, 103
fishing/fishermen, 6, 17, 42, 46, 48–50, 52, 56, 110, 126, 137, 141, 157, 164
flooding, 12–13, 41–45, 55–57, 84, 89–90, 102, 165n1; artificial, 38, 40
floodplains, 38, 41, 43–44, 55, 89
focus groups, 11, 13, 79–80, 104, 106, 112
Fonds Européens pour le Développement (FED), 44
food security, 38, 51–52, 56, 119, 123, 141, 148–149, 152, 163, 166n1

food stands, 42, 45, 51
Four Communes, 26–28, 165n3
French colonialism, 17, 20, 23, 25–29, 36–37, 40–41, 46, 101, 160
Fréquence-Terenga (radio station), 89
funerals, 13, 46, 103, 115

Gambia, 17, 21, 49–50, 52, 115, 126, 137, 164
Ganjool region, 5–7, 11–13, 15–16, 115; development in, 19, 38, 45–55, 143–157, 167n1; family decisions about serious illnesses in, 130–142; health strategies of residents in, 96, 102–103, 106; history of, 17, 37–38, 40, 45–57; mothers' concern for child health in, 124–129; politics of gender and household in, 18, 116–124. See also Daru-Mumbaay
garab u tubaab, 98. See also biomedicine
garab u wolof, 98, 112. See also Wolof medicine
gender, 6–8, 10–11, 101; and development in Ganjool, 151–152; division of labor, 55–56, 119; and global health reform, 72, 77–79, 82–83; mothers' concerns for child health, 124–129; politics of household, 18, 116–124. See also women
general assemblies, 73, 77, 86–87, 161
generation, 6, 11, 55–56, 124; and family decisions about serious illnesses, 18, 130–142
generic pharmaceuticals, 2, 5, 61, 79–81, 85, 91, 161. See also pharmaceuticals
germ theory of disease, 24
Get Ndar, 12, 23–24, 74, 76, 166n4
Global Fund for AIDS, Malaria, and Tuberculosis, 65, 68
global health reform, 2–5, 8–12, 19, 35, 58–63, 159–160, 164; and development in Ganjool, 155; efficiency-driven, 2, 8, 59, 62–63, 81; epidemiological profile of Senegal, 63–68, 66; equity-driven, 61–62; ethical frameworks for, 61–63; in Pikine, 17–18, 85–87, 94; in Saint Louis medical district, 17, 35, 68–83
global South, 2, 63
God, 108–114, 138–139; waiting for, 104, 111–114, 163–164
"Goorgoorlu," 167n4
Gorée, 25–26, 165n3
grand place, 14, 47, 54, 150, 153
gross domestic product (GDP), 3, 4, 59, 159
groundnuts, 25, 34, 42, 46
"Group of 77," 32
GTZ (German development agency), 44
Guinean therapeutic traditions, 98–100, 167n1
gum trade, 40

Haalpulaar families, 47, 151
habitus, 10
halal (acceptable), 109
haram (forbidden), 109
head doctor. See MC (médecin-chef de district)

head nurses (ICPs), 4–5, 11, 13, 43; epidemiological data from, 64; in Get Ndar, 166n4; and global health reform, 68–76, 78–80, 82, 88, 160, 166nn3,5; and health strategies of residents, 98, 102, 107–108, 111, 113; at Pikine health post, 56–57, 84–85, 87–95, 162, 166nn6,7

health clinics, 2, 4, 11–12, 45; epidemiological profile of, 63, 65; and global health reform, 58, 60–61, 68–72, 80, 82; and health strategies of residents, 97, 107–108. See also dispensaries; health posts

health committees, 11–12; and development in Ganjool, 154; in Get Ndar, 166n4; and global health reform, 61, 68–69, 71–79, 81–82, 159, 161, 166n2; in Pikine, 12, 76, 85–95

Health Development Index, 66

health huts/health hut workers, 6, 13, 47, 57, 68, 116–117, 124, 163; and childbirth, 152–154, 164; and development in Ganjool, 143–156, 164; and health strategies of residents, 103–107, 113

health infrastructure, 3, 19, 32, 45, 56, 67, 85, 154

health posts, 4–5, 12–13; and conflicts between medical personnel and local communities, 17–18; epidemiological data for, 64, 67; and global health reform, 58, 68–82, 160–161; and health strategies of residents, 97, 103, 107–108, 111; history of, 56–57; monitoring of, 75–76, 82, 166n3; in Pikine, 84–95, 166nn6,7; in Tassinère, 13, 57, 68, 103–104, 107–108, 126–127, 153. See also dispensaries; health clinics

Health Promotion Associations, 73. See also health committees

health resources, 5–6, 10, 13, 17, 19, 163; epidemiological profile of, 11, 65; and family decisions about serious illnesses, 18, 130–142; and global health reform, 59, 62–63, 69–74, 77, 79, 81; and mothers' concerns for child health, 124; in Pikine, 44–45, 86, 93

health strategies of residents, 6–7, 18–19, 96–108, 163

health talk (causerie), 146–148, 156

health worker (SUTSAS) strike, 64, 76, 161, 166n3

heart disease, 65

herbalism, 98, 100, 107, 109, 129, 133–134, 136

HIV/AIDS, 2–3, 6, 63, 65, 67–68, 102, 130, 146–148, 155–156, 162

home birth, 92, 104, 153

hospitals, 2, 12, 23–24, 57; and family decisions about serious illnesses, 133–134, 136, 138–139; and global health reform, 65, 78–80, 82; and health strategies of residents, 97, 104, 106–108, 111; and Pikine health post, 89–90

household census, 16, 102, 167–168n3

household heads, 146; and family decisions about serious illnesses, 130–142; and labor of male dependents, 6, 50–52, 56, 115, 132, 138, 140; and mothers' concerns for child health, 125–126, 128; and politics of gender and household, 117–118, 122–123, 167nn2,4

households, 4, 6, 8, 11, 13–14; expenses (see DQ); family decisions about serious illnesses, 18, 130–142, 162; mothers' concerns for child health, 124–129, 162; politics of gender, 18, 116–124. See also household heads

Human Development Index, 64

human rights. See right to health

hydroelectric power station, 31, 38

hypertension, 65, 79, 97–98, 102, 163

ICPs (infirmier-chefs de poste). See head nurses (ICPs)

illnesses, 4–6, 8–11, 13, 15, 18, 24; family decisions about serious illnesses, 18, 130–142; and global health reform, 56, 62; and health strategies of residents, 96–109, 111–113; and mothers' concerns for child health, 124–129; during sonsaa (red onion) season, 53–54

indigent status, 75, 85, 88

inequalities, social/political, 3–4, 6–7, 9–10, 17–18, 20, 162, 164; and development in Ganjool, 148, 154–155; and global health reform, 63, 76, 81–82, 160–161; and Pikine health post, 94

infant/child deaths, 3, 65–67, 66, 105, 107, 128–129

infectious diseases, 45, 65

informal labor market, 41–42, 44–45, 55–56, 83, 106

Information, Education, and Communication (IEC) campaigns, 155

information boycott, 64, 76, 166n3

Institut Pasteur (Tunisia), 24

International Monetary Fund (IMF), 32

interviews, 11–13, 15; about food security, 51–52; and global health reform, 58, 64, 79; and Pikine health post, 85–93

irrigation, 31, 38, 46, 49, 154

Islam, 6, 15, 20, 98; conversion to, 15; and family decisions about serious illnesses, 133–134, 136, 141; and health strategies of residents, 18, 97–98, 101–102, 106–107, 109–111, 113; history of in Senegal, 22, 35–36, 47; politics of gender and household, 118, 122

"Islam corner," 47

Islamic Conference, 32

Islamization, 101, 109

jakaa. See mosques

JAMRA (Muslim organization), 67–68

jëgg (transporting goods by camel), 48

jinne (evil spirit), 109

Jolof empire, 21

jumaa (Friday mosque), 47

kilifa. *See* authority figure
Koran, 103, 110–111, 118, 167n2

labor. *See* employment
labor histories, 48–49, 52
lambatu (to go back and forth), 100, 104, 111–113, 162
lay midwives, 83, 102
leviratic practice, 116
liberation theology, 63
life expectancy, 65
local officials, 3, 4, 5, 7, 10–11; and global health reform, 58, 61, 69–77, 160; history of in Senegal, 33–34, 37, 45; in Pikine, 17, 86, 89–91, 94. *See also* health committees; participatory management
loi cadre, and French colonial rule, 29
"lost decade," 159
lotissement. *See* zoning

malaria (sibiiru), 3, 13, 162–163; and development in Ganjool, 156; epidemiological data for, 65, 68; and family decisions about serious illnesses, 138–139; and global health reform, 79; and health strategies of residents, 102–103, 105–106, 108; history of in Senegal, 24, 45; and mothers' concerns for child health, 126, 127; and Pikine health post, 90
Mali, 23, 29, 31, 38, 167n2
malnutrition, 3, 65–66, 103, 105, 127, 146, 148–149, 156, 163, 167n2
Manantali dam, 31, 38, 40, 165n5
marabouts (Muslim leaders/scholars), 29, 102
marginalization, 3, 17, 43, 51, 81–82, 154, 164
mariage à la mode du pays (cohabitation), 23
market-based medical care, 3, 5, 10, 17, 159, 162; and global health reform, 59, 78, 80; and health strategies of residents, 96; in Pikine, 84–95
marriage, 49–50, 56, 116–128, 165n5, 167nn1,2; and brideprice, 49, 117, 167n1
Marxist critical theory, 9
massage, traditional, 1
maternal deaths, 3, 65, 66
maternal health, 65, 69, 161, 166n2
maternity wards, 68, 92, 156, 164
Mauritania, 23, 26–27, 38, 40, 47, 51
MC (médecin-chef de district; head doctor), 64, 69, 82; and global health reform, 69–71, 73–76, 82; and Pikine health post, 88–89, 91, 93, 162
measles, 65
medical districts, 11–12, 58–59, 160. *See also* Saint Louis medical district
medical personnel, 4–5, 11–13, 18, 45, 56; epidemiological data from, 64; and global health reform, 59, 61, 68–81, 160–161; in Get Ndar, 166n4; and health strategies of residents, 97–98, 107–108, 113; at Pikine health post, 84–85, 87–95
medical pluralism, 97–102, 104, 114

medicines. *See* pharmaceuticals
men's health practices, 13, 130–142, 162
métis (Creole) population, 23, 26, 28
microbusinesses, 42, 51, 106, 164
midwives: and global health reform, 65, 68–69, 71, 74, 78–79, 83, 161; and health strategies of residents, 102, 108; at Pikine health post, 85, 89, 93
migration, 6, 15, 126, 137–139, 141, 147, 167n2; history of, 35, 40–43, 46, 49–52, 55–57; illegal, 35, 56, 168n1; of young men, 8, 17, 35, 49–50, 56, 115, 157, 164
mill, diesel-operated, 47, 144, 155
millet, 46–47, 148
Ministry of Environment, 40
Ministry of Health, 6, 11–12, 15, 81, 101, 163, 166n5; and development in Ganjool, 145, 149; and global health reform, 61, 63, 70, 73, 76, 160; and health strategies of residents, 101–102
mocc (traditional healing technique involving massage and body manipulations), 1, 107, 111
mocckat (healer who practices mocc), 1, 98
modernity, European, 20, 25, 28
mokk pooj (femininity as marital bond), 123, 156
monitoring of health posts, 75–76, 82, 166n3
monopolies, 26
mool (fishermen), 49–50, 52. *See also* fishing/fishermen
mortality. *See* deaths
mosques, 44, 47, 136, 147
mosquitoes, 24
MSM (men who have sex with men), 67
Muid, 46–47, 143
multigenerational households, 117–118, 124–128
Mumbaay. *See* Daru-Mumbaay
municipal officials. *See* local officials
Murids, 25–27, 29, 31, 35, 165n4
Muslim leaders, 22, 27, 29
Muslims, 8, 15, 35–36, 67–68, 101–103, 106, 109–111, 165n1

nationalization, 30–31
Ndar-Tuut, 23, 70
ndëp (exorcism of traditional spirits), 101
négritude, 28–29, 36
neighborhood associations, 73, 77
neoliberalism, 2–4, 8–10, 19, 21; and global health reform, 58–59, 62, 80, 160; and health strategies of residents, 96; history of in Senegal, 17, 32–35, 37
Ngeyeen neighborhood, 13, 47, 116–129, 137, 167n3
NGOs (nongovernmental organizations), 4, 6, 15, 61, 68, 96, 102, 144–145, 167n1. *See also names of specific NGOs*
Niasse, Abdoulaye, 22
nivaquine, 106
Nkrumah, Kwame, 29
nuclear households, 118, 124, 126, 135

nurses. *See* head nurses (ICPs)
nurses' aides, 15, 68–69, 84, 98, 112
nutritional surveillance projects, 6, 145–149, 155–156, 166n2, 167n2
Nyerere, Julius, 29

obesity, 98, 166n1
older men. *See* household heads
onion farming, 37, 48–56, 105, 115, 131–132, 137–139, 141, 157, 167n1; and women, 1–2, 13, 50, 52–54, 125–127, 143, 158
oral rehydration therapy, 65, 103, 105, 127–128
Organisation pour la Mise en Valeur du Fleuve Sénégal (OMVS), 31, 38, 41, 57, 154
originaires (black Senegalese with French citizenship), 26–28
Ortner, Sherry, 7–8
Othering, 7–8, 16

parasites, 45
Partenariat Lille-Saint Louis, 89, 166n3
participant observation, 11, 13
participatory management, 2, 4, 17; and family decisions about serious illnesses, 142; and global health reform, 58, 69–77, 81–82; at Pikine health post, 85, 93–95, 161–162
Parti Démocratique Sénégalais (PDS), 30, 34, 89, 94
Parti Socialiste (PS), 34, 89, 94
patrilocal residence patterns, 117
patron-client relationships, 22, 29, 31, 34, 94
Peanut Basin, 25, 34, 42
peanut production/trade, 25, 30–31, 34, 40, 42, 46
peasants, 21, 25–26, 31, 38
People Living with AIDS, 3
perspectives, multiple, 4–5, 8–9, 11–12, 14, 17
pharmaceuticals, 2, 5, 14; abuse of access by medical personnel, 75–76, 87–88, 93; and development in Ganjool, 150–151; and family decisions about serious illnesses, 133; and global health reform, 60–61, 68–69, 71, 73–76, 78–82, 161, 166n2; and health strategies of residents, 101, 103, 106–108; at Pikine dispensary, 85–91, 93
Pikine, 5–7, 11–14, 16, 164; flooding in, 12, 84, 90; global health reform in, 78–79, 161; health committee in, 12, 76, 85–95; health post in, 84–95, 162, 166nn6,7; health strategies of residents in, 104, 106–108, 111–112; history of, 17, 37–38, 41–46, 55–57; market-based medicine in, 84–95
Pikine Development Association, 45
Pikine Project, 44
pilgrimages, 101, 109, 113
Plan International, 16, 144–145, 149–155, 167–168nn1,3
poliomyelitis vaccination, 143–144

polygyny, 18, 109, 116–117, 120–127
Pont Faidherbe, 23
population growth, 17, 23, 40–41, 43, 47, 64, 66, 85
postes de santé, 68. *See also* dispensaries; health posts
poststructuralists, 7
poverty, 2–3; and development in Ganjool, 148–149, 156; epidemiological data for, 64, 67; and global health reform, 59–60, 62–63, 71, 78, 81–82, 160–161; and health strategies of residents, 105–107, 111, 163, 166n1; history of in Senegal, 32, 34, 38, 40, 42, 51, 55; and mothers' concerns for child health, 128; in Pikine, 18, 85–86, 91–92
power relations, 5–7, 9, 11, 14, 18–19, 26, 35, 100, 145, 163. *See also* authority figure (kilifa)
practice theory, 7–8, 10
prayers, 14–15, 47, 53, 100, 109, 111–113, 129, 134, 136
prenatal care, 65, 67, 104
preventative strategies, 125, 129–131, 142, 162–163; and global health reform, 59–60, 78, 166n2; and health strategies of residents, 18, 96–98, 102, 104–105, 110, 112–114; for HIV/AIDS, 3, 67–68
primary health care (PHC), 3, 5, 59–61, 63–64, 69–70, 74, 81, 92, 103, 141, 161, 167n1
print media, 73, 89, 102, 113
privacy, 15–16, 123, 153–154, 156
privatization, 2; and global health reform, 17, 59–60, 70–71, 78–81; and health strategies of residents, 106; history of, 32, 34, 37, 42; at Pikine health post, 87
pseudonyms, 17
public fountains, 44

quality of care, 4–5, 18; and global health reform, 61, 69–70, 72, 76, 78–80, 82, 160; and health strategies of residents, 97, 108; at Pikine health post, 85, 93
quarantine, 24
quartier non-loti (unplanned neighborhoods), 43–44

rabb (ancestral spirits), 109–111
race, 10, 20, 26–27
radio news, 13, 89, 91, 102, 113, 117
railroads, 25, 46
rational economic actors, 6, 18, 96, 155, 163
redistributive justice, 62–63
red onions, 37, 48, 51–55. *See also* onion farming; sonsaa (red onion) season
reform. *See* global health reform
reproductive rights, 66, 166n1
respiratory infections, 65
responsibilization (making someone take responsibility), 2, 5; and development in Ganjool, 148–149; and family decisions about serious illnesses, 142; and global health reform, 59, 61, 70–72, 75–76, 81,

161; and health strategies of residents, 96, 98, 106, 113; at Pikine health post, 92
rice production, 31, 38
right to health, 5, 17, 59–60, 62
Rufisque, 26, 165n3
rural communities, 4–6, 8, 11–13, 55–57, 162; epidemiological profile of, 64, 67; and global health reform, 60, 68, 72, 82; and health strategies of residents, 98, 102–103, 106–107; history of, 20, 25, 29–31, 33–34, 37–38, 40–43, 45; mothers' concerns for child health in, 124–129; and Pikine health post, 92; and sonsaa (red onion) season, 1–2, 52–55, 115, 125, 131 (see also onion farming). See also Daru-Mumbaay; Ganjool region
rural flight, 17, 57

sabar (drum), 55
safety net provisions, 81, 85
Saint Louis, 4–5, 9, 26, 39, 165n3; global health reform in, 58–83; health practice in, 102–108; history of, 17, 22–26, 37–57, 39, 165n3
Saint Louis (city), 6, 9, 12, 15, 18; as "dry city," 40–45, 165n1; history of, 17, 22–23, 25–26, 37–38, 40–45; politics of, 70–72
Saint Louis medical district, 4, 11–12, 42, 160; and global health reform, 68–83; and Pikine health post, 85–86, 93–95; utility problem in, 70–72
salinization, 31, 37–38, 40, 48–49, 54
salt mines, 46
sanitation services, 38, 42–45, 56
schools, 6, 38, 43–44, 47–48, 86, 145, 149, 151–152. See also education
Seck, Mamadu, 76–77, 86–91, 166n4, 166n6
Senegal: epidemiological profile of, 63–68, 66; French colonialism, 17, 20, 23, 25–29, 36–37, 40–41, 46; history of, 20–36, 21, 38, 40, 46, 165nn4,6,7; independence (1960), 17, 26, 28–34, 36, 40–41, 57
Senegal River Valley, 21, 31, 38, 40–42, 49, 57, 154
Senghor, Léopold Sédar, 28–32, 165n6
senior men. See household heads
seriñ (Muslim cleric; healer), 102, 106–107, 109, 111–112
"serious games," 8, 10, 141
serious illnesses, 4, 79–80, 116, 162–163; family decisions about, 18, 130–142
seroprevalence rate, 67
sex education, 146–147
sexually transmitted infections (STIs), 146–148. See also HIV/AIDS
sex workers, 44, 56, 67
shantytowns (bidonvilles), 38, 41–43, 56, 165n2; health strategies of residents in, 106; market-based medicine in, 84–95; Pikine as, 5, 11, 17, 43–45, 84–95
sharia (Islamic law), 35, 167n2
sibiiru. See malaria
SIDA Service, 68
sister-city partnership, 145, 152, 166n3

slave trade, 21–22, 36
social capital, 7, 31, 77, 82, 138, 155
social contract, 5, 76
social justice, 63
Social Science and Medicine, 9
socioeconomic change, 4, 6, 15, 97, 101, 148–149, 154–155
sonsaa (red onion) season, 1–2, 52–55, 115, 125, 131. See also onion farming
Sor, 23–24
spirit possession, 102, 109–110
state-citizen partnerships, 5, 17, 58, 61, 76, 81, 142, 161
structural adjustment programs (SAPs), 2–3, 10, 159; and global health reform, 58–60, 63, 80; history of, 20–21, 32, 34
sub-Saharan Africa, 2, 19, 61, 65–66, 97–98
Sufi orders (tariqa), 20, 22, 25, 27, 29–30, 36, 101, 109, 160
SUTSAS (Syndicat autonome des travailleurs de la santé et de l'action sociale), 64, 76, 161, 166n3
suurga (strangers or foreigners), 51
suutuura (privacy or discretion), 16, 123, 154, 156

tariqa. See Sufi orders
tas (chronic tiredness), 131
Tassinère health post, 13, 57, 68, 103–104, 107–108, 126–127, 153
taxis, 89–90, 138–139
tea drinking, 3, 12–13, 52, 55, 79, 117, 133, 147
telephone service, 45
television, 102, 113
tension. See hypertension
theater troupe incident, 150–152, 155
tirailleurs Sénégalais (West African troops), 27
tooy (illness due to overwork and depletion), 131
total fertility rate (TFR), 66–67, 66
tourism, 38, 40, 42, 56, 115, 132
traders. See traveling merchants
trade slaves, 21–22
traditional medicine, 1, 6, 13, 97–101, 105–113, 133–134, 136–137. See also Wolof medicine
trash removal. See waste disposal
traveling merchants (bana-bana), 48, 51–52, 56
tubaabs (westerners), 104, 115, 150–151
tuberculosis, 3
tuul (protection against metal weapons), 110
tuur (tea drinking party), 55. See also tea drinking

UNESCO, 71
UNICEF, 60–61
Union Progressive Sénégalais (UPS) party, 30, 165n6
unions, 64, 76, 161, 166n3

United Nations, 30; International
  Conference on Population and
  Development, 66; UNICEF, 60–61
United States Agency for International
  Development (USAID), 65
Université Gaston Berger, 132
University of Saint Louis, 42, 132, 166n7
urban communities, 2–6, 8, 11–12, 55–57,
  162; epidemiological profile of, 67; and
  global health reform, 65, 67–68, 70, 78,
  81–82; health strategies of residents in,
  98, 102, 106–107, 166n1; history of, 17,
  20, 28, 33–34, 37, 40–45, 165n1; and
  Pikine health post, 92. See also Pikine;
  shantytowns (bidonvilles)
urbanization, 6, 38
urban planning, 41, 43–44
user fees, 2, 5; and global health reform,
  59–61, 68–70, 78–81, 161; and health
  strategies of residents, 106, 113; at Pikine
  health post, 85, 87, 91, 93
utilitarian frameworks, 62–63, 81

vaccinations, 24, 65, 68–69, 79, 101,
  143–144, 166n2
village chiefs, 46, 117, 150–152, 155,
  163–164
villages, 1–2, 5–6, 11, 13–16; and global
  health reform, 61, 68; health strategies of
  residents in, 102–114; history of, 41,
  45–52, 57; mothers' concerns for child
  health in, 116, 124–129; politics of gender
  and household in, 116–124. See also
  Mumbaay; Pikine; names of other villages

Waalo, 46, 48, 165n3
Wade, Abdoulaye, 30, 34–35, 165n7
Washington Consensus, 32
waste disposal, 11, 24, 42–45, 55–56
water, potable, 11, 24, 38, 43–45, 56, 70–72,
  166n2, 167n3
weddings, 13, 46, 54, 107, 115, 123
Western self, 7–8, 22
Weston, Kate, 14
widows, 116, 138, 167n2
witchcraft, 102, 133
Wolof kingdoms, 21–22, 46, 165nn3,4
Wolof language, 14–15, 103, 109, 112, 167n4

Wolof medicine, 18, 97–98, 101, 104,
  109–113, 125–126, 133. See also
  traditional medicine
Wolof society, 8, 11, 18, 22, 40, 47, 162,
  165n5; and development in Ganjool, 147,
  153; and family decisions about serious
  illnesses, 130–131, 133–134, 140–141;
  and health strategies of residents, 97–98;
  politics of gender and household in,
  118–128. See also entries beginning with
  Wolof
women, 4, 6, 13–14; and development in
  Ganjool, 143–148, 152–155; domestic
  work of, 50–51, 53–54, 56, 118–119,
  125–127, 167n3; employment of, 42, 45,
  50–51, 55–56, 106, 118–120, 122–124;
  and family decisions about serious
  illnesses, 130, 133, 135, 137–139, 142;
  and global health reform, 72, 77–79,
  82–83, 161; health strategies of, 12, 18,
  96–99, 101, 104–108, 111–113, 167n1; in
  microcommerce, 42, 51, 106; mothers'
  concerns for child health, 116, 124–129;
  and onion farming, 1–2, 13, 50, 52–54,
  125–127; and Pikine health post, 89, 91,
  94–95; politics of gender and household,
  116–124
women's groups, 12–13, 73, 106
World Bank, 32, 60, 62–63
"World Development Report: Investing in
  Health" (World Bank), 60
World Health Organization (WHO), 60–61,
  65
World Islamic Conference (2007), 34
World War I, 26–27
World War II, 28
wujj, 120–121. See also co-wives

Xaal Yoon Wi (Pikine women's group),
  12–13
xiiboon (sickly), 105, 149

yellow fever, 24
young men: and fishing, 17, 49; migration
  of, 8, 17, 35, 49–50, 56, 115, 157, 164;
  serious illnesses of, 18, 130–142, 162

zoning (lotissement), 37–38, 44–45

ABOUT THE AUTHOR

ELLEN E. FOLEY is an assistant professor of international development and social change in the Department of International Development, Community, and Environment at Clark University. Her research examines the intersection of global health policies and national health priorities with the community and household politics of managing ill health in marginalized communities. She has conducted research among African immigrants in Philadelphia and Worcester, analyzing health disparities and access to health resources, particularly access to HIV/AIDS prevention information, testing, and treatment. Her current research explores the social construction of gender and sexuality in the context of shifting marital patterns and transactional sex in urban Senegal. Professor Foley studied anthropology and women's studies at Kalamazoo College (B.A., 1994), and medical anthropology, the anthropology of development, and African studies at Michigan State University (Ph.D., 2002).

CPSIA information can be obtained at www.ICGtesting.com
Printed in the USA
267937BV00001B/91/P